The New
High Protein
Diet Cookbook

The New High Protein Diet Cookbook

Charles &
Maureen Clark

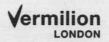

Vermilion
LONDON

3 5 7 9 10 8 6 4

Text © Charles and Maureen Clark 2003
Illustrations © Judy Stevens 2003.

First published in the United Kingdom in 2003 by
Vermilion, an imprint of Ebury Press
Random House UK Ltd
Random House
20 Vauxhall Bridge Road
London SW1V 2SA

Random House Australia (Pty) Limited
20 Alfred Street, Milsons Point, Sydney
New South Wales 2061, Australia

Random House New Zealand Limited
18 Poland Road, Glenfield
Auckland 10, New Zealand

Random House (Pty) Limited
Endulini, 5A Jubilee Road, Parktown 2193, South Africa

The Random House UK Limited Reg. No. 954009
www.randomhouse.co.uk
Papers used by Vermilion are natural, recyclable products
made from wood grown in sustainable forests

A CIP catalogue record for this book is available from the British Library

ISBN 0 09 1889707

Typeset by Palimpsest Book Production Limited,
Polmont, Stirlingshire

Printed and bound in Great Britain by
Bookmarque Ltd, Croydon, Surrey

The advice offered in this book is not intended to be a substitute for the
advice and counsel of your personal physician. Always consult a medical
practitioner before embarking on a diet or a course of exercise. Neither the
author nor the publishers can be held responsible for any loss or claim
arising out of the use, or misuse, of the suggestions made, or the failure to
take medical advice.

Contents

Acknowledgements

We thank our children, David and Heather, for their critical evaluation of the recipes in their evolutionary development, although perhaps next time they could be a little more diplomatic in their comments!

Special thanks to Sarah, Kate, Lesley and Julia at Ebury Press for their infinite patience and assistance, and especially to Fiona for her sound advice and unwavering support.

Further information can be obtained on:
www.charlesclark.uk.com

Dr Clark consults at:
The London Diabetes and Lipid Centre
14 Wimpole Street
London W1G 9SX
Tel: 020 7636 9901

Introduction

Have you ever wondered how some people seem to be able to eat as much as they like, and not put on an ounce in weight, but when you look at food you instantly gain 5 kilos? Well, you're about to find out! On this diet, you can eat unlimited amounts of delicious gourmet food, and lose weight at the same time. How? By using your brain to diet for you. You are going to use your body's own natural weight control mechanism to lose weight. You didn't know you had a 'weight control mechanism'? Well you do, you just have to adhere to a simple eating pattern, and you can eat virtually as much delicious food as you want, and lose all your excess fat. No counting calories, no rigid exercise regimes, and definitely no drugs. In fact the aim of this book is to show you how you can enjoy delicious food in virtually every normal situation and still diet successfully, with only one single restriction in your diet: that you reduce refined carbohydrates.

This is not like any diet you've ever tried before. You've been through the demoralizing experience of rigidly adhering to a daily 1000-calorie diet of polystyrene food, and the scales still refuse to budge. You've tried diets with high-fibre, low-calorie, low-fat, high-carbohydrate, detox . . . in fact, you've tried them all, and you're still the same weight. No longer! This time you will lose weight quickly, easily and healthily. You will not be hungry, and you won't need any willpower. This all seems too good to be true, but it's not. Providing you keep to the rules – which are simple

– you will be amazed at how easy it is to lose weight, feel well and look great!

The recipes in this book are based on the high-protein, low-carbohydrate diet described in *The New High Protein Diet*, on which many thousands of people have already lost weight easily. The principles of the diet are explained in *The New High Protein Diet* (published by Vermilion), but the main rule you cannot break is that you *must* restrict your carbohydrate intake to 40 grams per day. This stimulates the 'fat-burning' mechanism in your body (honestly, you do have one of these, and it does work) to use body fat preferentially as your main source of energy, and the kilos literally peel away. I would advise you to read *The New High Protein Diet* to understand how to apply the principles of this immensely successful diet to guarantee quick, easy and painless weight loss. To lose weight easily on a healthy, nutritious diet, you must follow these simple rules:

Restricted Foods

- Carbohydrates *must* be severely restricted to low levels
- Restrict fruit
- Alcohol: no beer, cider or fortified/sweet wines (sherry, port, Madeira)
- Avoid coffee, if possible; if not, have decaffeinated coffee
- Virtually no milk – even skimmed milk
- No fruit juices
- No pulses or grains in the early stage of the diet
- No carbonated soft drinks, except the 'diet' variety

Foods included in diet – virtually without restriction

- Virtually no restriction on the amount of protein
- Virtually no restriction on 'pure' fats

- Include eggs in your diet
- Include fresh vegetables
- Alcohol: dry wine (white or red) and spirits, in moderation
- Drink tea
- 'Diet' soft drinks only

General advice

- Stir-fry whenever possible
- Incorporate garlic and ginger in your diet
- Eat a substantial breakfast
- Eat an orange (or take a vitamin C supplement) every day
- Include herbs and spices in your diet
- Multivitamin supplements – one per day
- Regular exercise
- Measure shape before weight
- Vary your menu as much as possible

One of the main aims of this book is to provide you with relatively simple, nutritious gourmet meals which are suitable for the wide variety of different lifestyles which we all lead, in order that they may be applied to *real* life, rather than just for special occasions. Gourmet food – even gourmet 'diet' food – can be just as quick and simple to prepare as junk food, when you know how! And it's very important to maintain your nutrition whilst dieting; there is no point in looking better just to make yourself unwell. This diet will probably be the healthiest food you have ever eaten – whether on or off a 'diet'. A brief indication of the immense nutritional value of the meals is given in a preamble to many of the recipes, to convince you – if you need any further proof – of how healthy delicious food can be on a successful weight-losing diet.

Inevitably, the tremendous variety of different lifestyles enjoyed today means that we all have different needs and expectations from our diet, usually determined by the constraints of time. For most of us, there simply isn't enough time in the day to prepare healthy food, or so we are led to believe. This book will prove to you that there is enough time, with just a little preparation, to enjoy a healthy diet which will also ensure *healthy* and sustainable weight loss, without hunger. There is a recipe to suit every occasion in this cookbook, from light lunch to formal dinner party.

A word which recurs regularly in the book is 'antioxidant', but what exactly are antioxidants? Antioxidants mop up 'free radicals', which are electrons released during the trillions of chemical reactions which occur in our body every second. It all sounds very complicated (and it is), but the bottom line is that antioxidants keep us healthy, and seriously delay the ageing process, so we obviously have to include them in any healthy diet. Where do they come from? Basically, antioxidants occur in two main forms: either as proteins in the body (which we can manufacture from essential proteins in our diet), or as vitamins (especially vitamins A, C and E) and minerals present in a healthy diet which includes meat in any form (beef, lamb, pork), poultry, fish, shellfish, dairy produce, eggs, fresh fruit and vegetables, and nuts. So this diet has been specifically designed to make you healthy, as well as slim! Of course, it is possible to obtain all of our essential nutrients (except vitamin B12) from vegetables, but it is much more difficult, and only really suitable for those with a significant amount of time to devote to calculating the nutritional content of various vegetables.

Obviously, it's much easier to maintain a diet if your kitchen is well-stocked. This will solve the problem of selecting a recipe, then discovering you don't have all the necessary ingredients. The secret of a successful diet is a well-stocked kitchen, so every week check to ensure you have the following, and replenish when necessary. It doesn't take much time, it doesn't cost much, and it will make the difference between a successful diet, and just another failure!

- extra-virgin olive oil
- butter
- cheese(s), according to taste
- sour cream
- crème fraîche
- mayonnaise
- free-range eggs (large)
- fresh beef, poultry, pork, or lamb, according to taste
- fresh fish
- tinned tuna (preferably in brine)
- frozen prawns
- herbs (fresh and dried)
- garlic
- onions
- fresh vegetables, especially peppers (red, green and yellow, because they have different vitamin concentrations), carrots, broccoli and spring onions
- fresh ginger root
- oranges, lemons and limes
- fresh tomatoes
- tinned plum tomatoes
- black peppercorns
- shellfish
- tomato purée
- Dijon mustard
- tomato juice
- nuts – especially Brazil nuts, pine nuts and walnuts

To obtain the best nutrition (and flavour), *never overcook vegtables* as most of the essential nutrients (vitamins and minerals) will be lost during cooking. Nutrients leach out into water, so the most healthy (and practical) way to cook vegetables is by either steaming or stir-frying, which seals in the nutrients quickly. Steaming vegetables is a very simple and healthy method of cooking, with the advantage that the vegetables are effectively cooking while you can prepare the rest of the meal: ideal for the cook in a hurry! The vegetables are suspended in a perforated steaming compartment over (not in) a small volume of boiling water and the steamer covered. They cook quickly, retaining their texture, taste and nutrition; spinach, for example, takes only about 3 minutes. There are many varieties of simple, inexpensive steamers available, from circular, folding steamers that fit inside a saucepan, to Chinese bamboo steamers.

To summarize, the following is a general guide to foods included in or excluded from the diet:

Foods included virtually without restriction

Herbs and spices
Fish and shellfish
Meat and poultry
Oils and dressings
Sauces
Vegetables (except those with a high carbohydrate content, such as potatoes and parsnips)

Foods where some restrictions apply

Drinks
Dairy products
Eggs (up to two per day)
Fruit
Nuts
Soups

Foods excluded during the weight-loss phase

Biscuits, cakes and pastries
Bread, flour, grains and cereals
Desserts
Fast foods
Pasta and noodles
Rice
Snack foods

Keep within the unrestricted and partially restricted categories, and you will lose weight easily and healthily.

Read the labels on packaged foods to determine their carbohydrate content and, if you're uncertain, leave the food on the shelf.

Chapter 1

Morning Starters

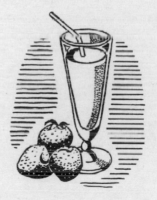

It is absolutely essential to have a healthy and satisfying breakfast if you really want to diet successfully. Unfortunately, there really is no alternative. We appreciate this is difficult for many people, because there doesn't appear to be enough time to prepare good tasty food whilst performing the myriad of other tasks that beset us in the morning: preparing the children's breakfast, getting the family ready for school, going to work . . . The list seems almost endless, but with a little forward planning it will not take much time to have that essential healthy breakfast, and complete all the remaining items of the morning routine.

But why is it so essential to have a satisfying breakfast for a diet to be successful? Surely it is more sensible *not* to eat if we are not hungry, especially as many of us don't have a substantial appetite first thing in the morning. Not so! A satisfying breakfast sets the controlling mechanism for your appetite for the rest of the day. If you set the controls wrongly in the morning, you end up snacking constantly (on fattening foods) for the rest of the day. Set the controls correctly, and you will have no desire to snack as you will not be hungry, and you will programme your hormones to burn your own body fat in preference to the calories in the food you eat.

And how do we achieve this minor miracle? Actually it is very simple indeed. Carbohydrates increase the production of a hormone called 'insulin' in the body. This hormone causes the body to make fat from the food we eat. If you reduce your carbohydrate intake to less than 40 grams per day, you reduce insulin production, so you *burn body fat and lose weight naturally*. Proteins and fats do not stimulate insulin production without carbohydrates, so if you restrict carbohydrates in your diet, *you can eat virtually unlimited amounts of other foods and still lose weight at about 2–3lbs per week*. Proteins and fats also slow your digestion of foods, so if you have a satisfying breakfast of these foods, and exclude carbohydrates, you won't be hungry because your food is absorbed more slowly.

Let's summarize so that you are completely clear on why it is absolutely essential to have a good, satisfying and healthy breakfast to ensure a successful, *real* weight-losing diet.

- Carbohydrates stimulate insulin production, which converts calories from food into fat. Omit refined carbohydrates from your diet, especially at breakfast, and you will start to burn your body fat *irrespective of the number of calories you eat*. In practice, this means no bread, toast, cereals, jams, marmalade, croissants (or pastries) for breakfast.
- If you eat proteins and fats and *less than 40 grams of carbohydrates* in your diet, your body will be programmed to burn body fat as a source of energy, and you will inevitably lose weight.
- Proteins and fats slow the digestion of food, so you don't feel hungry for longer, and there is no temptation to snack.

What types of food will provide a healthy satisfying breakfast, and are low in carbohydrates so they actually stimulate the fat-burning process?

- **Eggs**
  All methods of preparation: boiled, scrambled,
  poached, fried, baked, or as an omelette with various
  fillings (see page 21).

- **Meats**
  Ham, gammon, bacon (with eggs!), salami,
  kabanos . . .

- **Cheese**
  Virtually all varieties of cheese contain insignificant
  amounts of carbohydrates, so they are allowed
  without restriction in this diet.

- **Poultry**
  Pre-cooked chicken (legs, wings, breast), either
  prepared the previous evening, or purchased from
  the supermarket. Pre-packed slices of chicken breast.

- **Mushrooms**
  Grilled on a single slice of buttered wholemeal toast
  is a delicious, and satisfying, start to the day. A
  single slice of bread is only 15–17 grams of
  carbohydrate, so it won't ruin the diet. Always butter
  the toast; the fat in the butter will slow your
  digestion and prevent hunger pangs mid-morning.

- **Tomatoes**
  Once again, grilled tomatoes on a single slice of
  buttered wholemeal toast is delicious, especially if
  you sprinkle over some finely chopped fresh herbs,
  such as oregano or basil. And tinned tomatoes have
  even more of the essential antioxidant lycopene than
  the fresh variety.

- **Fish**
  Fish can provide such a simple, quick and nutritious
  meal for breakfast. Grilled or jugged kippers, poached
  haddock or pre-cooked mackerel take minutes to
  prepare, and provide a very satisfying breakfast.

A healthy breakfast doesn't take up much time in the morning, with just a little preparation. It is very simple, and very quick, to prepare poached or scrambled eggs in the microwave, to boil eggs (perhaps hard-boiled and mixed with mayonnaise with some chopped tomato, or basil, coriander, diced spring onion), grill gammon, grill mushrooms or cheese on a single slice of toast, grill kippers, or have a continental breakfast of sliced cold meat, ham or salami, with cheeses, boiled eggs, or even some pre-cooked chicken.

The recipes for preparing the quick and tasty breakfasts above are explained in *The New High Protein Diet*. Of course, if you have a little more time, perhaps at the weekend, breakfast can become much more interesting, with recipes as varied as savoury crêpes to Halloumi and pancetta kebabs. The recipes in each chapter are not exclusively restricted to that particular chapter or, for that matter, to a specific time of day. There are major overlaps between the different sections of the book. This is particularly relevant to morning starters, which may be equally applicable to light lunch, or quick-and-easy meals.

Savoury Crêpes

Crêpes are virtually pure carbohydrate, so how can we possibly include them in a low-carbohydrate diet? Very easily! This diet is based upon common sense principles. As each crêpe only contains about 5–6 grams of carbohydrate (and less carbohydrate if made with water instead of milk) you can see that providing you have no more than 2–3 savoury crêpes for breakfast (which will be more than sufficient with the delicious and satisfying fillings), you are well within the carbohydrate limit for the day.

For 4–5

100 grams plain flour
pinch of salt
1 large free-range egg, beaten
300 ml full-cream milk (or water)
1 tbsp melted butter

Some prefer to use milk for sweet crêpes and water for savoury crêpes. We use full-cream milk for all crêpes, but if you want to reduce carbohydrate intake further, you can use water instead of milk. The above ingredients make about 16 crêpes. The carbohydrate content of crêpes made with milk is approximately 6 grams per crêpe; with water it is about 5 grams per crêpe, so the difference is virtually insignificant. This recipe can be made by hand, or using a blender.

* Mix together the flour and salt, then sieve the mixture into a medium bowl.
* Add the beaten egg, whisking constantly.
* Gradually blend in the milk, drawing the mixture to the centre of the bowl until you achieve an even consistency.
* Allow to stand for 1 hour before making the crêpes.
* Just before cooking, stir in the melted butter to the mixture.

Crêpes can be made either by the traditional method, or by using a commercial crêpe-maker. The latter is relatively inexpensive, and provides a very quick and easy way of crêpe-making.

Traditional method
* Add a level tbsp of butter to a medium, non-stick frying pan, melt the butter over medium heat, and evenly coat the pan.
* Add 2 tbsp of the mixture to the pan, then tip the pan to evenly coat the base of the pan.

- Cook for about 20–30 seconds, then remove with a palette knife.

Crêpe-maker

- Pour the mixture into a wide, shallow dish.
- Turn on the crêpe-maker. When hot, dip the crêpe-maker horizonally onto the mixture to lightly coat, then allow the crêpe to cook. When the edge of the crêpe is lightly browned, remove with a palette spatula and repeat the process.

Savoury crêpes can be presented in several ways: either folded into triangles and topped with the savoury filling, folded in half over the filling, or rolled around the selected filling.

Pancetta and Egg Crêpes

For 2

6 crêpes (as above)
4 medium free-range eggs
6 thin slices of pancetta
freshly ground black pepper
1 tbsp chopped fresh basil

- Prepare the crêpes (page 17).
- Poach (or scramble) the eggs to taste.

At the same time

- Grill the pancetta until crispy.
- Fold the crêpes into triangles, and place three on each plate.
- Top with the eggs and crispy pancetta.
- Season with freshly ground black pepper, and garnish with chopped fresh basil.

CARBOHYDRATE CONTENT PER SERVING: 18 GRAMS

Haddock and Parmesan Crêpes

For 2

1 medium haddock fillet (approximately 150 grams)
200 ml full-cream milk
15 grams unsalted butter
15 grams plain flour
1 tbsp chopped fresh flat-leaf parsley
pinch of rock salt
freshly ground black pepper
6 crêpes
2 tbsp freshly grated Parmesan cheese

- Place the haddock fillet in a shallow oven-safe dish, pour over 50 ml of milk, and cover with pierced aluminium foil.
- Bake in the centre of a pre-heated oven at 180°C (gas 4) for 15–18 minutes.
- Remove from the oven and allow to cool, then flake lightly.

At the same time

- Prepare the crêpes (page 17).
- Melt the butter in a medium saucepan, remove from the heat and stir in the flour.
- Return to a low heat and gradually blend in the milk.
- When the sauce begins to thicken, stir in the flaked haddock and the chopped parsley.
- Season to taste.
- Spoon the mixture evenly over the crêpes, then fold the crêpes in half.
- Transfer the crêpes to a grill-safe dish, top with the Parmesan cheese, and grill under a pre-heated moderate grill (no closer than 8 cm from the grill) until the cheese begins to brown, then serve immediately.

CARBOHYDRATE CONTENT PER SERVING: 24 GRAMS

Mushroom and Chicken Crêpes

For 2

1 tbsp extra-virgin olive oil
100 grams small button mushrooms, halved
   lengthways
6 crêpes
15 grams unsalted butter
15 grams plain flour
150 ml full-cream milk
1 tbsp chopped fresh basil
100 grams pre-cooked chicken breast, chopped into
   small cubes
pinch of rock salt
freshly ground black pepper

- Heat the virgin olive oil in a small saucepan, and lightly sauté the mushrooms.

At the same time

- Prepare the crêpes (page 17).
- Melt the butter in a medium saucepan, remove from the heat and stir in the flour.
- Return to a low heat and gradually blend in the milk.
- When the sauce begins to thicken, stir in the mushrooms, chicken and the chopped basil.
- Season to taste.
- Spoon the mixture evenly over the crêpes, then fold the crêpes in half, and serve immediately.

CARBOHYDRATE CONTENT PER SERVING: 26 GRAMS

Omelette

Omelettes can be simple or . . . simple, but whatever
the filling (or lack of filling), omelette is always a
perfect meal, because fresh free-range eggs are both
nutritious and delicious.

For 2

4 fresh, large free-range eggs
2 tbsp full-cream milk
pinch of rock salt
freshly ground black pepper
30 grams unsalted butter

- Beat the eggs in a medium mixing bowl, add the
  milk, and season to taste.
- Heat the butter in a medium omelette pan, add the
  egg mixture, and allow to cook on high for about a
  minute, then gently lift the edges of the omelette
  with a spatula, allowing the egg to cook more
  rapidly.
- When the egg just begins to set, but is still creamy,
  fold the sides of the omelette to the centre, and
  serve immediately.

Of course there are many fillings for omelette; here are
a few suggestions:

- Parma ham (diced), diced plum tomato and chives
- Chopped fresh basil and coriander
- Freshly grated Gruyère and chives, garnished with
  freshly grated Parmesan
- Asparagus and basil
- Finely chopped cooked chicken breast with tarragon
- Diced smoked salmon with dill
- Diced and deseeded red and yellow peppers, with
  $1/2$ deseeded finely chopped medium green chilli
  (optional)

- Sliced mushrooms (pre-cooked) with chopped tomato and chopped fresh oregano.

CARBOHYDRATE CONTENT PER SERVING: 1–4 GRAMS
(DEPENDING ON FILLING)

Halloumi with Pancetta Kebabs

For 2

100–150 grams of Halloumi cheese, cubed
8 vine-ripened cherry tomatoes
6–8 rashers of pancetta
1 tbsp chopped fresh coriander leaves
fresh coriander, to garnish

- Soak 4 wooden skewers for 2 hours before use (preferably overnight).
- Divide the cheese into small cubes. Halloumi is a firm cheese, so this is relatively easy.
- Thread the cubes of cheese and cherry tomatoes alternately on the skewers, and grill under a medium grill (8–10 cm from the grill) for 4–5 minutes, turning once.

At the same time

- Lightly grill the pancetta for 3–4 minutes, turning once.
- Top with chopped fresh coriander and serve the kebabs and pancetta immediately, garnished with sprigs of fresh coriander.

CARBOHYDRATE CONTENT PER SERVING: 5 GRAMS

Eggs with Herbs and Tomatoes

For 2

1 tbsp extra-virgin olive oil
1 small red onion, peeled and diced
1 medium garlic clove, peeled and chopped finely
200 gram tin of plum tomatoes, drained and chopped
1 tbsp chopped fresh coriander
1 tbsp chopped fresh flat-leaf parsley
1 tbsp chopped fresh oregano (or ½ tsp dried
   oregano)
2 large free-range eggs
freshly ground black pepper

- Heat the extra-virgin olive oil in a medium frying pan and sauté the onion and garlic for 2–3 minutes.
- Stir in the tomatoes and herbs, and simmer gently for 12–14 minutes.
- Crack the eggs separately over the herb tomatoes, in each of the four quadrants of the pan.
- Cook for 4–5 minutes.
- Season with freshly ground black pepper, and serve immediately.

CARBOHYDRATE CONTENT PER SERVING: 5 GRAMS

Breakfast Tortilla

For 2

4 large eggs (preferably free-range)
2 tbsp full-cream milk
freshly ground black pepper
25 grams butter
1 tbsp chopped fresh basil
1 tbsp chopped fresh chives
2 slices Parma ham, chopped finely
pinch of rock salt
2 medium flour tortillas

handful of wild rocket leaves
2 small vine-ripened tomatoes, diced

Scrambled eggs can be made by the traditional method, or more quickly using a microwave oven. Both methods are described.

Traditional method

- Break the eggs into a mixing bowl, add the milk and a little freshly ground black pepper, and beat gently with a fork to an even consistency.
- Melt the butter in a small pan over a low heat, and add the eggs.
- Stirring constantly, move the edge of the mixture to the middle with a circular motion, for about 2–3 minutes.
- Remove from heat just before the eggs have set to allow the heat of the pan to gently finish the cooking, stir in the basil, chives and Parma ham, and season to taste.

By microwave

- Add the beaten eggs to a microwave-safe bowl and place in the centre of the microwave oven.
- Set on 'high' and cook for 1 minute. Remove the bowl from microwave, and stir mixture, bringing the edges to the centre.
- Return to microwave and cook on 'high' for another minute, and repeat. Repeat the process for another minute, or until the mixture has not quite set.
- Stir in the basil, chives and Parma ham, and season to taste.

At the same time

- Wrap the tortillas in aluminium foil, and warm in a hot oven for 1 minute.

- Place half of the wild rocket leaves and chopped tomato on each tortilla, top with the scrambled egg mixture, and season with freshly ground black pepper.
- Close the tortilla, and serve immediately.

CARBOHYDRATE CONTENT PER SERVING: 23 GRAMS
(INCLUDING 20 GRAMS FOR THE TORTILLA)

Bagel Delights

Bagels are a 'forbidden' food, as they contain a high carbohydrate content. Of course, this is just a general rule to help you reduce your carbohydrate intake. The average bagel contains about 30 grams of carbohydrate, so you can have ½ a bagel, as an open sandwich, without any problems for your diet. The secret of this diet is *moderation* of refined carbohydrates in your diet, and virtually unlimited quantities of other foods, almost all of which are very healthy!

Emmental and Prosciutto Bagel

For 2

1 medium bagel, halved horizontally
6 thin slices of Prosciutto ham
75 grams of Emmental cheese, sliced thinly
1 tbsp freshly chopped chives
freshly ground black pepper

- Lightly toast the bagel halves for no more than 30 seconds.
- Top each half with slices of Prosciutto ham then Emmental cheese.
- Toast the bagels until the cheese begins to melt.
- Sprinkle over the chopped chives, season to taste and serve immediately.

CARBOHYDRATE CONTENT PER SERVING: 15 GRAMS

Sun-dried Tomatoes and Herbs Bagel

For 2

4 medium sun-dried tomatoes, sliced thinly
$1/2$ tbsp chopped fresh oregano
$1/2$ tbsp chopped fresh basil
freshly ground black pepper
1 medium bagel, halved horizontally
drizzle of extra-virgin olive oil

- Mix together the sun-dried tomatoes, oregano and herbs, and season to taste.
- Lightly toast the bagel halves for no more than 1 minute.
- Top with the tomato and herb mixture, and drizzle over a little extra-virgin olive oil, then serve immediately.

CARBOHYDRATE CONTENT PER SERVING: 20 GRAMS

Spinach and Mackerel Bagel

Mackerel is an excellent source of the omega-3 fatty acids, which are so essential for health. It can be purchased pre-cooked from delicatessens and supermarkets: the perfect *healthy* fast food.

For 2

1 medium mackerel, pre-cooked
1 tbsp mayonnaise
1 medium bagel, halved horizontally
75 grams fresh spinach
1 tbsp chopped fresh dill

- Flake the mackerel, and mix with a tbsp of mayonnaise.

At the same time

- Lightly toast the bagel halves for no more than 1 minute.
- Butter the bagel halves, and place the spinach leaves on each half.
- Top with the mackerel mayonnaise, sprinkle over the dill, and serve immediately.

CARBOHYDRATE CONTENT PER SERVING: 16 GRAMS

Breakfast Platter

A delicious breakfast platter can be simple or diverse, according to taste. Almost all of the foods can be purchased ready-to-eat (except boiled eggs, which only take a few minutes), and therefore this has to be the ultimate fast breakfast. And, as all of the foods contain virtually no carbohydrates (apart from fruit), you can virtually eat as much as you wish and still lose weight. A typical selection of appropriate foods would include:

- 'Pure' cooked meats, such as sliced ham, turkey, chicken or beef
- 'Prepared' cooked meats, such as virtually all of the continental salamis and sausages
- Virtually all natural cheeses. The only exceptions are some processed cheeses.
- Pre-cooked fish, such as mackerel
- Hard-boiled eggs
- Smoked salmon
- Pre-cooked chicken: legs, thighs, or breast
- Nuts: restrict to 50 grams, especially cashews, chestnuts, almonds and peanuts
- One piece of fruit, but definitely no bananas, which are very high in carbohydrates. For example, apples and oranges contain about 10–13 grams of carbohydrate each, compared with 30 grams in a banana!

Gammon with Mushrooms and Tomatoes

A healthy *dieting* breakfast doesn't need much time in the morning, just a little forethought and preparation. The secret, once again, is in shopping: keeping the *right* ingredients in your kitchen cupboards (see page 5) instead of the same old 'fast' breakfast ingredients, like cereals, bread, jams, marmalade and croissants. This meal is a perfect example of how you can eat healthily, and quickly, in the morning. And because this is a very flexible diet (apart from the absolute restriction on refined carbohydrates) you can vary the diet according to individual taste. So, for example, if you don't like gammon, or mushrooms, or tomatoes, just omit one of these from the meal. It will still be healthy and nutritious, because all of the ingredients are healthy in different ways (unlike most refined carbohydrates).

For 2

2 medium gammon steaks
2 tbsp extra-virgin olive oil
2 medium plum tomatoes, chopped
50 grams of chestnut mushrooms, wiped and halved
2 spring onions, chopped
1 tbsp chopped fresh basil
freshly ground black pepper

- Grill the gammon steaks under a medium grill for 4–5 minutes, turning once.

At the same time

- Heat the virgin olive oil in a medium saucepan, and sauté the tomatoes, mushrooms and spring onions for 2–3 minutes.
- Stir in the basil, and cook for a further minute.
- Serve the vegetables on the gammon steak, and season to taste.

CARBOHYDRATE CONTENT PER SERVING: 6 GRAMS

Toasted Cheese

There are endless variations on the theme of toasted cheese – the variety of cheese in itself is almost infinite – so the choice is yours; with high-quality food like cheese, the taste is inevitably superb.

For 2

2 slices of wholemeal bread
1 large plum tomato, sliced
50 grams of freshly grated cheese (try Wensleydale, Edam, Jarlsberg, Orkney, Emmental or Halloumi)
1 tsp Worcestershire sauce
freshly ground black pepper

- Lightly toast 1 side of the wholemeal bread.
- Arrange the slices of tomato on the other side, sprinkle over the cheese and drizzle over a few drops of Worcestershire sauce.
- Season with freshly ground black pepper, and lightly grill until the cheese melts and begins to turn golden.

CARBOHYDRATE CONTENT PER SERVING: 18 GRAMS

Breakfast Drinks

Although it really is essential to keep to the limit of 60 grams of carbohydrate per day for successful slimming, you can use foods with natural carbohydrates (such as fruits) providing you have virtually no refined carbohydrates in the day (especially bread). Effectively you are trading your bread ration for fruit, which is a much healthier option. The following recipes are for delicious and healthy juices, which provide the perfect start to any morning.

To enjoy fruit and vegetable juices, you really need to invest in a juicer, which separates the juice from the fibre. Many fruit juices are perfect on their own; blending juices simply adds to the natural flavours, and obviously increases your intake of healthy vitamins and minerals. Although it is not necessary to add water to natural juice, this has many advantages, as fluid intake is essential for health, and pure clean water is still the healthiest fluid ever 'invented'. The combinations of juices and water are merely intended as a guide; we all have different individual tastes, and you should vary the combination according to your own taste. For example, if you prefer your juice more dilute, add more water, and vice versa. But be careful not to exceed the quantities of fruit, as fruit is relatively high in carbohydrate per unit weight, and if you increase the amount of fruit you may inadvertently ruin your diet! A standard apple or orange contains about 13 grams of carbohydrate; of course this varies according to the actual size of each item, so the carbohydrate quantities per serve are necessarily approximate.

Citrus Stinger

Citrus fruits are particularly high in the essential antioxidant vitamin C.

For 2

1 medium grapefruit, peeled
2 medium oranges, peeled
1 tbsp freshly squeezed lime juice
50 ml water (optional)

* Juice the fruit and blend together.

CARBOHYDRATE CONTENT PER SERVING: 13 GRAMS

Watermelon Delight

Pure juice: deliciously refreshing. A rich source of vitamin A and folic acid.

For 2

Large slice of fresh watermelon
  (approximately 200 grams), skin removed
50 ml water

* Juice the watermelon and add water, to taste.

CARBOHYDRATE CONTENT PER SERVING: 7 GRAMS

Apple and Strawberry Appetizer

Apples and strawberries provide our total daily requirements of the antioxidant vitamins A and C.

For 2

1 medium apple
100 grams of fresh strawberries
100 ml water (optional)

- Juice the apple.
- Add apple juice to fresh strawberries in a blender, and blend together.
- Add water, to taste.

CARBOHYDRATE CONTENT PER SERVING: 10 GRAMS

Citrus Carrot

A perfect nutritional combination of vitamin A from carrots and vitamin C from oranges and lemons.

For 2

2 large carrots, washed and peeled
2 large Seville oranges, peeled
2 tbsp freshly squeezed lemon juice
50 ml water (optional)

- Juice the carrots and orange, and blend together with the lemon juice.
- Dilute with water, to taste.

CARBOHYDRATE CONTENT PER SERVING: 10 GRAMS

Raspberry and Apple Energizer

Calcium for strong bones and teeth, and potassium for a healthy heart, are both provided by this delicious juice.

For 2

I medium apple
100 grams of raspberries
100 ml water

- Juice the apple.
- Blend the apple juice with the raspberries.
- Dilute to taste.

CARBOHYDRATE CONTENT PER SERVING: 8 GRAMS

Berry Zest

This is the perfect tonic to prevent colds as it is so high in vitamin C.

For 2

100 grams blueberries
100 grams strawberries
1 tbsp freshly squeezed lime juice
100 ml water

* Blend together the blueberries, strawberries and lime juice.
* Dilute to taste.

CARBOHYDRATE CONTENT PER SERVING: 10 GRAMS

Kiwi Surprise

Rich in folic acid, which is essential for our blood cells to function efficiently.

For 2

3 kiwi fruit
1 large pear
50 ml water

* Juice and blend the kiwi fruit and pear.
* Dilute to taste.

CARBOHYDRATE CONTENT PER SERVING: 20 GRAMS

Tomato Juice

An excellent source of the antioxidant 'lycopene'.

For 2

4 large vine-ripened tomatoes
dash of Worcestershire sauce

- Juice the tomatoes.
- Stir in a dash of Worcestershire sauce.

CARBOHYDRATE CONTENT PER SERVING: 7 GRAMS

Mango and Strawberry Milkshake

This contains vitamins A and C from the fruits, and calcium and vitamin D from the milk.

For 2

1 mango
100 grams of ripe strawberries
125 ml cold full-cream milk

- Juice the mango.
- Blend together the mango juice, strawberries and milk.

CARBOHYDRATE CONTENT PER SERVING: 14 GRAMS

Blueberry Milkshake

Once again, a perfect combination of vitamin C from the fruit, and calcium and vitamin D from milk.

For 2

150 grams fresh blueberries
200 ml cold full-cream milk

- Juice the blueberries.
- Blend with the milk.

CARBOHYDRATE CONTENT PER SERVING: 16 GRAMS

Chapter 2

Soups

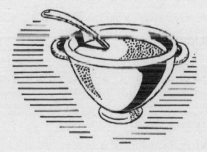

Soups are the ultimate meal: they can be prepared in advance, consumed hot or cold (obviously depending on the selection of soup), and are equally suitable for lunch, as a prelude to dinner, or a late-night supper on a cold winter evening. Most soups are relatively quick to prepare and are relatively inexpensive – and all the soups in this book are incredibly nutritious.

Pumpkin and Coriander Soup

A delicious soup with the marvellous antioxidant properties of coriander – which has also been known for centuries to protect against infection. Perfect to warm you up in winter, or as a light lunch.

For 2

2 tbsp extra-virgin olive oil
1 medium onion, peeled and diced
750 grams pumpkin, peeled and chopped
1½ tsp ground cumin
½ tsp ground turmeric
400 ml chicken stock
1 tbsp chopped fresh coriander
2 slices of fresh ginger root, peeled and chopped
    finely
pinch of salt
freshly ground black pepper
100 ml cream
1 tbsp chopped fresh chives

- Heat the extra-virgin olive oil in a large saucepan and sauté the onion and pumpkin for 2–3 minutes.
- Stir in the cumin and turmeric, and sauté for a further 2 minutes
- Add the chicken stock, coriander and ginger, bring to the boil, and simmer for 20–25 minutes.
- Transfer to a food processor and purée, then return to the saucepan.
- Season to taste, stir in about 80 ml of cream, and heat gently. Do not boil!
- Serve immediately with a swirl of cream, and garnish with freshly chopped chives.

CARBOHYDRATE CONTENT PER SERVING: 15 GRAMS

Borscht

There are many regional variations of this soup from Russia. Based unusually on beetroot, which provides an excellent supply of both folate and iron, this soup was popular across the social spectrum, from peasants to the Russian royal family!

For 2

15 grams unsalted butter
1 medium brown onion, peeled and diced finely
1 small garlic clove, peeled and chopped finely
3 small raw beetroot (about 500 grams), peeled and grated
500 ml beef stock
pinch of salt (depending on 'saltiness' of beef stock)
freshly ground black pepper
2 tsp freshly squeezed lemon juice
3 tbsp dry sherry
50 ml single cream

- Heat the butter in a large saucepan and sauté the onion and garlic for 2–3 minutes.
- Add the beetroot and stock, and season to taste.
- Bring to the boil, then lower the heat, cover, and gently simmer for about 40 minutes.
- Blend the mixture in a food processor, add the lemon juice and sherry to the soup, stir well and chill in the fridge for at least 3–4 hours.
- Serve chilled, adding a swirl of cream just before serving.

CARBOHYDRATE CONTENT PER SERVING: 25 GRAMS

Chilled Leek and Potato Soup

This includes one of our 'forbidden fruits', potato, which, of course, is not forbidden – in moderation! The recipe provides an excellent source of potassium, vitamin C, and the B vitamins thiamin (B_1) and pyridoxine (B_6).

For 2

50 grams unsalted butter
400 grams leeks, trimmed and sliced finely
1 medium potato, peeled and sliced finely
500 ml chicken stock
pinch of rock salt
freshly ground black pepper
100 ml single cream
1 tbsp chopped fresh basil

- Melt the butter in a medium saucepan, cover, and gently sweat the leeks and potato for about 10 minutes.
- Stir in the stock, season to taste and gently simmer for 15–20 minutes.

- Set aside to cool, then purée in a food processor.
- Immediately before serving, stir in the cream and check the seasoning.
- Garnish with chopped fresh basil.

CARBOHYDRATE CONTENT PER SERVING: 16 GRAMS

Creamy Gruyère Soup

This delicious soup combines the essential nutrients of calcium and vitamin D from the cheese with the healthy antioxidant properties of garlic and onion.

For 2

25 grams unsalted butter
1 medium brown onion, peeled and diced finely
1 garlic clove, peeled and chopped finely
1 tbsp plain flour
350 ml chicken stock
75 ml medium white wine
75 grams Gruyère cheese, grated finely
pinch of rock salt
freshly ground black pepper
100 ml single cream
chopped fresh chives and a swirl of cream, to
    garnish

- Melt the butter in a medium saucepan and gently sauté the onion and garlic for 2–3 minutes.
- Remove from the heat and stir in the flour.
- Stir in the stock gradually, return to the heat, bring to the boil, then reduce the heat and gently simmer for 5 minutes.
- Add the wine, season to taste, and simmer gently for about 20 minutes.
- Blend in the cheese, and heat through gently until the cheese melts.

- Purée the soup, and return to the heat.
- Stir in the cream, check the seasoning, and heat through gently.
- Serve immediately with a swirl of cream, and garnish with chopped fresh chives.

CARBOHYDRATE CONTENT PER SERVING: 13 GRAMS

Lemon and Chicken Soup

Lemon and chicken are a perfect gastronomic combination. The sharpness of the lemon is absorbed to perfection by the texture of the chicken. Apart from providing all of our essential amino acids from chicken, this recipe is also a rich source of the powerful antioxidants vitamin C from lemon juice and vitamin A from carrots.

For 2

30 grams of unsalted butter
1 medium brown onion, peeled and diced
1 medium carrot, peeled and grated
1 large ready-cooked chicken breast
   (approx 150 grams), chopped
3 tbsp freshly squeezed lemon juice
1 bay leaf
400 ml chicken stock
1 tbsp dry sherry
pinch of rock salt
freshly ground black pepper
100 ml single cream
swirl of cream, to garnish

- Melt the butter in a large saucepan and gently sauté the onion and carrot for 2–3 minutes.
- Add the chicken, lemon juice, bay leaf, stock and sherry, and season to taste.

- Bring to the boil, then reduce the heat and simmer gently for about 45 minutes.
- Remove the bay leaf, and purée the soup in a food processor.
- Stir in about 80 ml of cream and heat through gently.
- Serve immediately with a swirl of cream.

CARBOHYDRATE CONTENT PER SERVING: 8 GRAMS

Creamy Spinach and Coriander Soup

The nutritional value of spinach has been immortalized by Popeye, but with good reason. Spinach is an excellent source of iron, vitamins C and E, folate and potassium – proving conclusively that cartoons really are good for your health!

For 2

250 grams of spinach
400 ml chicken (or vegetable) stock
2 tbsp extra-virgin olive oil
1 medium onion, peeled and diced
1 garlic clove, peeled and chopped finely
2 tsp plain flour
1 tbsp chopped fresh coriander
pinch of rock salt
freshly ground black pepper
100 ml single cream
chopped fresh chives and a swirl of cream, to
    garnish

- Add the spinach to the stock in a medium saucepan and bring to the boil.
- Reduce the heat and gently simmer for about 5 minutes.
- Set aside to cool.

- Heat the extra-virgin olive oil in a medium frying pan and gently sauté the onion and garlic.
- Remove from the heat and stir in the flour.
- Gradually blend in the stock (including spinach), add the coriander, and season to taste.
- Simmer gently for 4–5 minutes then purée in a food processor.
- Return the soup to a clean saucepan, stir in about 80 ml of cream and heat through gently.
- Serve immediately, garnished with chopped fresh chives and a swirl of cream.

CARBOHYDRATE CONTENT PER SERVING: 15 GRAMS

Broccoli and Basil Soup

Broccoli is so healthy it's difficult to know where to begin. A rich source of folate, iron, calcium, zinc and the antioxidants vitamins C, E and beta-carotene, the inclusion of broccoli is essential to a healthy diet.

For 2

25 grams of butter
1 medium brown onion, peeled and diced
1 small garlic clove, peeled and chopped finely
500 ml chicken stock
250 grams of broccoli florets
2 tbsp chopped fresh basil
pinch of rock salt
freshly ground black pepper
swirl of cream, to garnish

- Melt the butter in a large saucepan and sauté the onion and garlic for 2–3 minutes.
- Add the chicken stock and slowly bring to the boil.
- Stir in the broccoli florets and basil, season to taste, and gently simmer for 15–20 minutes.

- Remove from the heat and allow to cool.
- Blend in a food processor to a smooth purée and check the seasoning.
- Heat through before serving with a swirl of cream.

CARBOHYDRATE CONTENT PER SERVING: 3 GRAMS

French Onion Soup

Onions are included in many recipes, not only for their marvellous taste and texture, but also for their incredible nutritional properties. A naturally rich source of B vitamins and potassium, the antibacterial effect of onions has been recognized for centuries, and their potential benefits in lowering cholesterol and high blood pressure are becoming more generally accepted.

For 2

50 grams butter
5 medium brown onions, peeled and sliced
1 garlic clove, peeled and chopped finely
1 tsp brown sugar
1 tsp white wine vinegar
1 tbsp plain flour
450 ml beef stock
1 tsp chopped fresh flat-leaf parsley
1 tsp chopped fresh chives
pinch of rock salt (if necessary)
freshly ground black pepper
freshly grated Parmesan cheese and chopped fresh
    chives, to garnish

- Melt the butter in a medium saucepan and gently sweat the onions and garlic for about 15 minutes.
- Stir in the vinegar and sugar and sauté for a further 1–2 minutes.
- Remove from the heat and stir in the flour.

- Gradually stir in the stock, parsley and chives, and season to taste.
- Bring to the boil, then reduce the heat to a gentle simmer for 5–10 minutes.
- Serve immediately, garnished with freshly grated Parmesan cheese and chopped chives.

CARBOHYDRATE CONTENT PER SERVING: 22 GRAMS

Watercress Soup

Watercress has been known for centuries as a 'tonic' to improve health, but only recently have we established the incredibly high level of nutrients in this seemingly innocuous plant. With substantial amounts of carotenes, and vitamins C and E, watercress provides an excellent source of antioxidants and the essential nutrients calcium, folate, iron and potassium. And watercress soup tastes delicious!

For 2

25 grams of unsalted butter
1 small onion, peeled and diced
150 grams of watercress, finely chopped
250 ml chicken stock
150 ml full-cream milk
pinch of rock salt
freshly ground black pepper
1 tbsp freshly grated Parmesan cheese
swirl of single cream, to garnish

- Melt the butter in a medium saucepan and gently sauté the onion.
- Stir in the watercress, cook for 2–3 minutes until softened, then stir in the stock and milk.
- Heat through, and season to taste.
- Gently simmer for about 8–10 minutes.

- Stir in the Parmesan cheese.
- Remove from heat and purée the soup.
- Serve with a swirl of fresh single cream.

CARBOHYDRATE CONTENT PER SERVING: 7 GRAMS

Chapter 3

Light Lunch

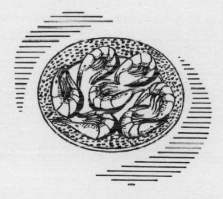

Lunch for most of us is dictated by the practical necessities of our lifestyle, and is therefore, by definition, 'light'. The days of heavy three- or four-course lunches are all but gone (thank goodness) because a substantial proportion of the meals were carbohydrates: bread, potatoes and sweet desserts at lunchtime are guaranteed to stimulate fat production by our metabolism.

Lunch should be tasty, nutritious, satisfying and attractive. This final attribute seems unusual, but it is actually one of the most important of all; unattractive, boring, tasteless meals lead to inevitable 'snacking' later in the day. The diet fails and, even worse, your nutritional intake is compromised, leading to a gradual impairment in health.

Even if you don't have time to prepare lunch on a regular basis, keep to the guidelines and you will still lose weight easily and healthily. The importance of this diet is that it is flexibly designed to adapt to your lifestyle, not the other way around.

Many of the following recipes are equally successful as light and delicious suppers.

Crab Soufflé

Soufflé is seldom considered a 'simple' or quick dish to prepare, but it is! Shellfish soufflés – of all varieties – are delicious, and incredibly healthy. Apart from its many other healthy qualities, crabmeat is an excellent source of zinc, a mineral essential for the function of the body's natural antioxidant enzymes.

For 2

3 large free-range eggs, separated
25 grams butter
25 grams plain flour
$1/2$ tsp dry mustard powder
2–3 drops of Tabasco sauce
150 ml full-cream milk
150–200 grams fresh white crab meat, cooked then
    chopped
1 tbsp chopped fresh dill
pinch of rock salt
freshly ground black pepper
sprigs of fresh dill, to garnish
150 grams of asparagus

- Separate the eggs, beat the yolks, and whisk the whites until firm.
- Melt the butter in a small saucepan.
- Add the flour and milk, stirring constantly until the mixture is smooth.
- Remove from the heat and allow to cool for 2–3 minutes, stirring occasionally.
- Stir in the mustard powder, Tabasco sauce, chopped crabmeat, dill and egg yolks, and season to taste.
- Beat in 1 tbsp of egg white to the mixture, then gradually 'fold' the remainder of the egg whites into the mixture.

- Lightly butter a soufflé dish and gently spoon in the mixture evenly.
- Bake in the centre of a pre-heated oven at 190°C (gas 5) for 25–30 minutes. (Ovens vary; the deciding factor is whether the soufflé has risen, but don't open the oven to find out, or the soufflé will definitely collapse!)

Just before the souffle is ready

- Lightly steam the asparagus.
- When the soufflé is ready, garnish with sprigs of fresh dill, and serve with the asparagus.

CARBOHYDRATE CONTENT PER SERVING: 14 GRAMS

Spicy Pork Patties

Hot and nutritious, but this recipe is equally enjoyable without the chilli, if you prefer.

For 2

3 tbsp extra-virgin olive oil
1 medium red onion, peeled and chopped finely
1 garlic clove, peeled and chopped finely
$^1/_2$ green chilli, deseeded and chopped finely
200 grams lean pork, minced
2 tsp Worcestershire sauce
1 egg white, beaten
freshly ground black pepper
chives and pepper salsa (page 257)

- Heat 1 tbsp of extra-virgin olive oil in a small saucepan and sauté the onion, garlic and chilli for 1–2 minutes.
- Allow to cool, then mix together the onion, garlic, chilli, pork, Worcestershire sauce and egg white, and season to taste.

- Form the mixture into 2 large patties, and cool in the fridge for 30–40 minutes.
- Heat the remaining olive oil in a frying pan, and cook the patties for 9–10 minutes, turning once.

At the same time

- Prepare the chives and pepper salsa.
- When ready, serve the spicy patties with the salsa.

> CARBOHYDRATE CONTENT PER SERVING: 13 GRAMS
> (INCLUDING SALSA)

Barbecue Turkey Salad

Rocket is an ancient aphrodisiac, so enjoy your meal!

For 2

2 tbsp extra-virgin olive oil
2 skinless turkey breasts, approximately
   100–125 grams each
100 grams wild rocket leaves, washed
1 tsp chopped fresh coriander
4 semi-dried tomatoes with herbs (page 254)
8–10 black olives, halved
freshly ground black pepper
50 ml French vinaigrette (page 266)
freshly grated Parmesan cheese

- Flatten the turkey breasts using a rolling pin, and brush with olive oil.
- Barbecue over medium heat for 8–10 minutes, turning once.
- Allow to cool, then slice across the diagonal into 1–2 cm strips.
- Mix together the char-grilled turkey, rocket leaves, coriander, semi-dried tomatoes, and black olives in a medium bowl.

- Season to taste, and toss with the vinaigrette.
- Garnish with shavings of freshly grated Parmesan cheese, and serve immediately.

CARBOHYDRATE CONTENT PER SERVING: 7 GRAMS

Lamb Cutlets with Herb Butter Sauce

This is a delicious light lunch (or supper), and is so simple and quick to prepare.

For 2

2 tbsp extra-virgin olive oil
6 medium lamb cutlets
75 grams unsalted butter
1 tbsp chopped fresh chives
1 tbsp chopped fresh rosemary
1 tsp Dijon mustard
freshly ground black pepper
75 grams broccoli florets
75 grams yellow squash
sprigs of fresh basil, to garnish

- Brush the cutlets on both sides with extra-virgin olive oil, and cook under a hot grill, or on a hot barbecue, for 6–7 minutes, turning once.
- Lightly steam the broccoli and squash.
- Heat the butter in a small saucepan, stir in the mustard and herbs, and season to taste.
- Serve the cutlets with the herb butter sauce and vegetables, garnished with fresh basil.

CARBOHYDRATE CONTENT PER SERVING: 7 GRAMS

Scrambled Eggs with Basil and Chervil

The potential combinations with scrambled eggs, as with omelettes, are almost infinite and limited only by your imagination and taste, but the following combination is particularly delicious – and simple.

For 2

50 grams unsalted butter
2 medium plum tomatoes, diced
1 spring onion, chopped finely
1 small garlic clove, peeled and chopped finely
2 tsp chopped fresh basil
2 tsp chopped fresh chervil
4 large free-range eggs, beaten
pinch of rock salt
freshly ground black pepper
2 tsp chopped fresh coriander

- Melt the butter in a medium frying pan and gently sauté the tomatoes, spring onion and garlic for 2–3 minutes.
- Add the basil, chervil and egg mixture, season to taste, and cook over medium heat, stirring frequently.
- When almost set, but still creamy, serve immediately, garnished with chopped fresh coriander.

CARBOHYDRATE CONTENT PER SERVING: 4 GRAMS

Mozzarella Chicken

This delicious meal is ideal for light lunch or supper. And incredibly healthy: protein from chicken and Mozzarella, lycopene and vitamin A from tomato, antioxidants *par excellence* from the coriander and chives . . . the list is endless.

For 2

2 skinless chicken breast fillets,
    approximately 100–125 grams each
25 grams butter, cubed
1 large vine-ripened tomato, sliced thickly
1 tbsp chopped fresh chives
2 tsp chopped fresh coriander
4–6 thin slices of Mozzarella cheese
freshly ground black pepper
75 grams of wild rocket
passata vinaigrette (page 268)
fresh coriander leaves, to garnish

- Flatten the chicken fillets and place in a medium
  baking dish. Dot with cubes of butter, cover with
  pierced aluminium foil, and cook in the centre of a
  pre-heated oven at 180°C (gas 4) for 35–40 minutes.
- Remove the chicken fillets with a perforated spoon
  and transfer them to a grill tray.
- Top with slices of tomato, sprinkle over the herbs,
  and add a final layer of thin slices of Mozzarella.
- Grill under a hot grill (approximately 8–10 cm from
  the grill) until the cheese has melted.
- Serve on a bed of wild rocket, drizzle over a little
  passata vinaigrette, and garnish with fresh coriander
  leaves.

CARBOHYDRATE CONTENT PER SERVING: 4 GRAMS

Creamy Prawns with Basil

Cayenne chilli originated in India (unlike other chillis
which were introduced to Europe by Christopher
Columbus from his travels in the west), but cayenne
actually takes its name from a region of French
Guyana! Confusing, but incredibly nutritious.

For 2

3 tbsp extra-virgin olive oil
1 spring onion, chopped finely
1 garlic clove, peeled and chopped finely
300 grams cooked prawns, thawed
4 tbsp water
1 tbsp dry sherry
1 tsp Dijon mustard
1 tbsp chopped fresh basil
1 tsp cornflour
100 ml single cream
pinch of cayenne pepper
sprigs of fresh dill, to garnish

- Heat the extra-virgin olive oil in a wok and stir-fry the spring onion and garlic for about a minute.
- Add the prawns and stir-fry over medium heat for another minute.
- Stir in 2 tbsp water, sherry and mustard.
- Mix the cornflour with 2 tbsp water to a smooth paste.
- Remove the pan from the heat, and gradually stir in the cornflour paste.
- Return to the heat and simmer gently for 1–2 minutes, then stir in the cream and cayenne pepper.
- Heat through gently, and serve immediately, garnished with sprigs of fresh dill.

CARBOHYDRATE CONTENT PER SERVING: 5 GRAMS

Salmon Steaks with Leek and Lemon Butter Sauce

Once again, taste and nutrition are often inextricably linked. The superb nutrition from salmon, lacking only vitamin C, with the vitamin C from citrus fruits. Nature has a unique way of ensuring our continued good health; this is the real fast food.

For 2

leek and lemon butter sauce (page 274)
2 salmon steaks, approximately 125–150 grams each
freshly ground black pepper
3 tbsp extra-virgin olive oil
sprigs of fresh dill, to garnish
green salad with herbs (page 252)

- Prepare the leek and lemon butter sauce, and set aside
- Brush the salmon with extra-virgin olive oil on both sides and season with freshly ground black pepper.
- Grill under a medium grill for 4–5 minutes per side.
- Pour over the leek and lemon butter sauce.
- Garnish with fresh dill, and serve with green salad with herbs.

CARBOHYDRATE CONTENT PER SERVING: 4 GRAMS
(INCLUDING SALAD)

Beefburgers with Chilli and Tomato Sauce

This contains vitamins A and C from chillis and tomatoes, the powerful antioxidant lycopene from tomatoes, and antioxidants from onion and garlic. Can you believe that beefburgers could ever be this healthy?

For 2

3 tbsp extra-virgin olive oil
3 spring onions, chopped finely
1 garlic clove, peeled and chopped finely
200 grams lean beef mince
2 tsp chopped fresh oregano
freshly ground black pepper

1 egg white, beaten
sprigs of fresh oregano, to garnish

- Heat 1 tbsp of extra-virgin olive oil in a small saucepan and lightly sauté the spring onions and garlic for 1–2 minutes.
- Allow them to cool.
- Mix together the spring onions, garlic, mince and oregano, season to taste, and bind together with the egg white.
- Form into 2 burgers, and cool in the fridge for 30–40 minutes.
- Heat 2 tbsp extra-virgin olive oil in a frying pan, and cook the burgers for about 10 minutes, turning once.
- Garnish with sprigs of fresh oregano, and serve with chilli tomato sauce (page 275), and crispy green salad (page 248).

CARBOHYDRATE CONTENT PER SERVING: 7 GRAMS
(INCLUDING SALAD AND CHILLI SAUCE)

Basil Pesto Turkey with Char-grilled Vegetables and Sesame Seeds

This is a delicious light lunch, full of healthy nutrition. Pine nuts are an excellent source of vitamin B_1 and vitamin E with the dietary advantage of a relatively low carbohydrate content.

For 2

basil pesto sauce (page 276)
200 grams turkey breast fillet, sliced
char-grilled vegetables with sesame seeds (page 229)
fresh oregano leaves, to garnish

- Prepare the pesto sauce according to the recipe on page 276.

- Coat the slices of turkey breast with pesto sauce and marinate for 3–4 hours.
- Place on a grill tray under a medium grill, approximately 8 cm from the heat, and grill for 8–10 minutes, turning once.

At the same time

- Char-grill the vegetables.
- Serve the basil pesto turkey with char-grilled vegetables, garnished with fresh oregano leaves.

CARBOHYDRATE CONTENT PER SERVING: 14 GRAMS
(ONLY 2 GRAMS WITHOUT VEGETABLES)

Smoked Haddock Soufflé

This recipe includes essential amino acids and fatty acids from fish, calcium and vitamin D from milk, and folate and vitamin B_{12} from eggs. Being healthy never tasted so good!

For 2

100 grams smoked haddock
250 ml full-cream milk
1 bay leaf
3 large free-range eggs, separated
25 grams butter
25 grams plain flour
1 tbsp chopped fresh basil
pinch of rock salt
freshly ground black pepper
1 tbsp chopped fresh dill, to garnish
rocket and olive salad (page 247)

- Place the haddock in the base of a baking dish, then pour 100 ml of milk around the fish and add the bay leaf.

- Cover with pierced aluminium foil, and bake in the centre of a pre-heated oven at 180°C (gas 4) for 10–12 minutes.
- Remove the haddock with a draining spoon, allow to cool, and flake the haddock.
- Separate the eggs, beat the yolks, and whisk the whites until thickened.
- Melt the butter in a small saucepan, then stir in the flour and remaining 150 ml of milk, stirring constantly until the mixture is evenly thickened.
- Remove from the heat and allow to cool for a couple of minutes, stirring occasionally.
- Season to taste, then stir in the egg yolks and flaked haddock.
- Gradually 'fold' the egg whites into the mixture.
- Lightly butter four individual soufflé dishes and gently spoon in the mixture evenly.
- Place the soufflé dishes on a baking tray and bake in the centre of a pre-heated oven at 190°C (gas 5) for 25–30 minutes. (Ovens vary; the deciding factor is whether the soufflé has risen and is lightly browned.)
- Soufflé must be served immediately, or it will collapse! Garnish with chopped fresh dill and serve with rocket and olive salad.

CARBOHYDRATE CONTENT PER SERVING: 16 GRAMS
(INCLUDING SALAD)

Lamb with Spices

Cinnamon is an ancient remedy for colds. Both cinnamon and ginger are believed to have potent qualities to combat infection.

For 2

2 tsp ground coriander
2 tsp ground cumin

$^1/_2$ tsp ground turmeric
$^1/_2$ tsp ground cinnamon
pinch of cayenne pepper
pinch of rock salt
3 tbsp extra-virgin olive oil
250 grams lamb fillet, sliced thinly
3 spring onions, chopped into 4–5 cm lengths on the
    diagonal
2 slices of fresh ginger root, peeled and chopped
    finely
75 grams of mangetout
75 grams broccoli florets
100 grams button mushrooms, wiped and halved
1 tbsp dry sherry
2 tsp chopped fresh coriander
freshly ground black pepper
fresh coriander leaves, to garnish

- Mix together the ground spices in a medium bowl and coat the lamb.
- Heat 2 tbsp of extra-virgin olive oil in a wok and stir-fry the lamb for 3–4 minutes.
- Remove the lamb with a perforated spoon and set aside.
- Heat the remaining olive oil in the wok and stir-fry the spring onions, ginger, mangetout, broccoli, and mushrooms for 2–3 minutes.
- Add the sherry and coriander, return the lamb to the wok, and season to taste.
- Cook for a further 2 minutes and serve immediately, garnished with fresh coriander leaves.

CARBOHYDRATE CONTENT PER SERVING: 5 GRAMS

Scallop and Calamari Salad

Shellfish are such a healthy food, why restrict yourself to only one! The flavours of different shellfish merge beautifully together, and are particularly enhanced by garlic and ginger. This recipe provides an excellent source of iron, and all the essential amino acids.

For 2

30 grams butter
4 large scallops
2 tbsp extra-virgin olive oil
1 tsp sesame oil
2 garlic cloves, peeled and chopped finely
2 slices of fresh ginger root, peeled and chopped finely
8 raw tiger prawns, peeled and deveined (tails on)
200 grams fresh calamari tubes, chopped into 1 cm rings
100 grams mixed wild rocket and red oak lettuce
4 spring onions, chopped finely
1 tbsp chopped fresh coriander
freshly ground black pepper
oriental vinaigrette (page 268)
lime wedges

- Melt the butter in a small saucepan.
- Separate the corals from the scallops, slice the scallops into rounds horizontally, and gently sauté the scallops (and corals) for 3–4 minutes.
- Remove them from the pan with a perforated spoon, cover and set aside.
- Heat the olive oil and sesame oil in a wok and sauté the garlic and ginger for a minute.
- Add the prawns and calamari, and stir-fry for 2–3 minutes.
- Add the cooked scallops and heat through gently for about a minute.

- Toss the wild rocket, red oak lettuce, spring onions and coriander, season to taste, and transfer to plates.
- Arrange the scallops, prawns, and calamari on the salad, drizzle over the dressing, and serve with lime wedges.

CARBOHYDRATE CONTENT PER SERVING: NEGLIGIBLE

Baked Bolognese Peppers

Parmesan cheese tops this delicious meal perfectly, in more than just flavour. The vitamin D from cheese supplies the missing vitamin from this otherwise superbly nutritious dish.

For 4

2 tbsp extra-virgin olive oil
2 medium red onions, peeled and diced
2 garlic cloves, peeled and chopped finely
300 grams lean minced beef
1 tbsp tomato purée
4 large vine ripened tomatoes, peeled and diced (or a 400 gram tin of plum tomatoes, drained before use)
1 tbsp chopped fresh oregano
freshly ground black pepper
4 large red peppers, deseeded and top removed
freshly grated Parmesan cheese
fresh oregano, to garnish

- Heat the extra-virgin olive oil in a frying pan and sauté the onion and garlic for 1–2 minutes.
- Add the mince and stir until browned.
- Mix in the tomato purée, tomatoes and oregano, season to taste, and gently simmer for 6–8 minutes.
- Spoon the mixture into the peppers, and place the peppers on a baking tray, adding a little water to the tray.

- Cook in the centre of a pre-heated oven at 160°C (gas 2) for 30–35 minutes.
- Remove from the oven, and sprinkle freshly grated Parmesan cheese over the peppers.
- Grill under a medium grill until the cheese melts, garnish with fresh oregano, and serve immediately with semi-dried tomatoes with herbs (page 254).

CARBOHYDRATE CONTENT PER SERVING: 17 GRAMS

Smoked Trout Frittata

Smoked trout, fresh dill and fresh chives – what a perfect combination!

For 2

4 large free-range eggs, beaten
1 smoked trout, flaked and bones removed
1 tbsp chopped fresh dill
1 tbsp chopped fresh chives
pinch of rock salt
freshly ground black pepper
2 tbsp extra-virgin olive oil
sprigs of fresh dill, to garnish
100 grams of wild rocket

- Mix together the eggs, smoked trout, dill and chives, and season to taste.
- Heat the extra-virgin olive oil in a medium frying pan and pour in the egg mixture.
- Cook over low heat for about 10 minutes, without stirring.
- When almost set, place under a grill for 2–3 minutes until just set.
- Garnish with sprigs of fresh dill and serve immediately on a bed of wild rocket.

CARBOHYDRATE CONTENT PER SERVING: NEGLIGIBLE

Barbecued Turkey Keftas with Cucumber Raita

Spicy herb turkey keftas are simple and quick to prepare and cook, with just a little forethought. Cucumber raita adds a delicious cooling influence to the meal, and is also very high in essential nutrients, as cucumber is a rich source of potassium and sulphur.

For 2

350 grams of turkey breast, minced
1 medium onion, peeled and grated
1 garlic clove, peeled and chopped finely
1 tbsp chopped fresh basil
1 tbsp chopped fresh coriander
1 tsp paprika
1 egg white, separated
pinch of rock salt
freshly ground black pepper
3 tbsp extra-virgin olive oil
cucumber raita (page 281)

- Mix together the turkey, onion, garlic, basil, coriander, paprika and egg white, and season to taste.
- Mould the mixture to form a sausage shape around kebab sticks, pressing firmly, then cool in the fridge for 3–4 hours (to retain the kebabs' shape whilst barbecuing).
- Remove the kebabs from the fridge, brush with extra-virgin olive oil, and barbecue (or grill) on high for 6–7 minutes, turning once. Serve with cucumber raita.

CARBOHYDRATE CONTENT PER SERVING: 8 GRAMS
(INCLUDING RAITA)

Tuna with Creamy Herb Sauce

Mushrooms complement any healthy diet as a rich source of potassium, iron and vitamin B. Button mushrooms are particularly useful in a low-carbohydrate diet, as they have less carbohydrate than other varieties.

For 2

3 tbsp extra-virgin olive oil
3 shallots, peeled and chopped
1 garlic clove, peeled and chopped finely
50 grams of button mushrooms, trimmed, wiped, and halved
200 gram tin of tuna (in brine or springwater), drained
2 tsp chopped fresh dill
2 tsp chopped fresh basil
2 tsp chopped fresh flat-leaf parsley
pinch of rock salt
freshly ground black pepper
200 ml single cream
200 grams of spinach
fresh flat-leaf parsley and a pinch of paprika, to garnish

- Heat the extra-virgin olive oil in a medium frying pan and gently sauté the shallots and garlic for 2–3 minutes.
- Add the mushrooms and sauté over medium heat for a further 2 minutes.
- Stir in the tuna and herbs, and season to taste.
- Cook for another minute, then stir in the cream and heat through gently.

At the same time

- Lightly steam the spinach for 2–3 minutes.
- Serve immediately on a bed of lightly steamed spinach.
- Garnish with fresh flat-leaf parsley and a pinch of paprika.

CARBOHYDRATE CONTENT PER SERVING: 5 GRAMS

Egg Mayonnaise with Smoked Salmon

This recipe provides essential amino acids and essential omega-3 fatty acids from salmon, essential proteins and vitamin B from eggs, and even more antioxidants from herbs.

For 2

4 large free-range eggs, hard boiled and chopped finely
1 tbsp mayonnaise
1 tbsp chopped fresh basil
50 grams of smoked salmon, sliced finely
freshly ground black pepper
6 thin slices of French bread, freshly toasted and buttered
chopped fresh chives, to garnish

- Mix together the eggs, mayonnaise, basil and salmon, and season with freshly ground black pepper (no salt; smoked salmon is salty!).
- Spoon over the buttered French bread, and garnish with chopped fresh chives.

CARBOHYDRATE CONTENT PER SERVING: 19 GRAMS
(2 GRAMS WITHOUT BREAD)

Shellfish with Bok Choy

Tomatoes, especially when cooked, provide a rich source of lycopene, a powerful antioxidant. Together with the selenium and zinc (which are essential minerals required by the body to produce its own antioxidants) from shellfish, this is a powerful recipe to clear free radicals from the body, and stay healthy.

For 2

100 ml dry white wine
50 ml water
4 small fresh scallops, corals removed and sliced into
  rounds
2 tbsp extra-virgin olive oil
8 raw tiger prawns, shelled and deveined
1 garlic clove, peeled and chopped finely
3 large plum tomatoes, chopped
1 tsp tomato purée
2 tsp chopped fresh basil
1 tsp chopped fresh oregano
freshly ground black pepper
2 bok choy, halved vertically
fresh oregano leaves, to garnish

- Mix together the white wine and water in a small saucepan, then gently poach the scallop rounds (not the corals) for about 8 minutes.
- Heat the extra-virgin olive oil in a wok and stir-fry the prawns for 2 minutes.
- Add the scallop corals, garlic, tomatoes, tomato purée, and herbs.
- Season to taste and cook over medium heat for a further 2 minutes.

At the same time

- Lightly steam the bok choy for 3–4 minutes.
- Add the scallop rounds to the tomato and herb mixture, stir gently and heat through for about a minute.
- Serve immediately with lightly steamed bok choy, garnished with fresh oregano.

CARBOHYDRATE CONTENT PER SERVING: 6 GRAMS

Chilli Mayonnaise Turkey with Mangetout

This dish is just as delicious with normal mayonnaise
(page 268), garlic mayonnaise (page 269), herb
mayonnaise (page 269), or creamy curry mayonnaise
(page 271); it simply depends on individual taste. The
carbohydrate content is the same for all.

For 2

4 tbsp extra-virgin olive oil
350 grams of turkey breast fillet, sliced thinly
50 ml chilli mayonnaise (page 270)
50 grams of French beans
100 grams of mangetout
3 spring onions, chopped finely
1 garlic clove, peeled and chopped finely
2 slices of fresh ginger root, peeled and chopped
  finely
pinch of rock salt
freshly ground black pepper

* Prepare the mayonnaise according to the recipe you
  prefer.
* Heat 2 tbsp of extra-virgin olive oil in a wok and stir-
  fry the turkey breast for 4–5 minutes.
* Remove from the wok, pat dry and allow to cool.
* Mix the turkey breast with the mayonnaise.
* Heat the remaining 2 tbsp of virgin olive oil in the
  wok and stir-fry the French beans for 3–4 minutes.
* Add the mangetout, spring onions, garlic and ginger.
* Season to taste and stir-fry for 3–4 minutes.
* Serve immediately with the turkey and mayonnaise.

CARBOHYDRATE CONTENT PER SERVING: 4 GRAMS

Salmon with Watercress and Mint Sauce

Once again, the aphrodisiac qualities of the meal may have to be taken into account as much as the nutrition and taste. Mint has been recognized as an aphrodisiac for centuries, including by William Shakespeare no less!

For 2

watercress and mint sauce (page 283)
2 salmon fillets (approximately 150 grams each)
pinch of rock salt
freshly ground black pepper
green salad with herbs (page 252)
pinch of paprika

- Prepare the watercress and mint sauce, and set aside to chill in the fridge for 2–4 hours before serving.
- Place the salmon fillets in a shallow oven-safe dish (in a single layer), cover with pierced aluminium foil and cook in the centre of a pre-heated oven at 180°C (gas 4) for 15–20 minutes.
- Season to taste, and serve immediately with chilled watercress and mint sauce and green salad with herbs, garnished with a pinch of paprika.

CARBOHYDRATE CONTENT PER SERVING: 5 GRAMS
(INCLUDING SAUCE AND SALAD)

Crab and Herb Salad

This is one of the easiest salads to prepare, and one of the most delicious. It really is important to buy good ingredients whenever possible. If you can cook a fresh crab, please do so. We can't, so we always purchase crab ready-cooked! Tinned crab meat is almost as nutritious as fresh, so you can prepare this simple and delicious meal very quickly with just a little forethought when shopping. Remember, the secret of successful dieting is shopping!

For 2

1 large crab, cooked
100 grams mixed green lettuce leaves (frisee, green
    oak leaf, coral, mizuna and rocket)
1 tbsp chopped fresh basil
1 tbsp chopped fresh chives
1 tsp chopped fresh coriander
pinch of rock salt
freshly ground black pepper
honey and orange vinaigrette (page 267)
finely chopped spring onions and fresh basil leaves,
    to garnish

- Toss the mixed green lettuce leaves, basil, chives and coriander in a large salad bowl and season to taste.
- Remove the crab meat from the shell and arrange on the salad, separating the white and dark meat.
- Drizzle over the dressing, and garnish with finely chopped spring onions and fresh basil leaves.

CARBOHYDRATE CONTENT PER SERVING: NEGLIGIBLE
(WITH 'NORMAL' VINAIGRETTE – PAGE 266); 7 GRAMS
(WITH HONEY AND ORANGE VINAIGRETTE)

Lamb Burgers

Carrots are an excellent source of beta-carotene, a powerful antioxidant, which is also essential for night vision.

For 2

300 grams of lean lamb fillet, minced
1 tbsp chopped fresh coriander
1 tbsp chopped fresh basil

1 tbsp chopped fresh flat-leaf parsley
1 large carrot, peeled and grated finely
4 spring onions, chopped finely
1 garlic clove, peeled and chopped finely
1 large free-range egg, beaten
pinch of rock salt
freshly ground black pepper
watercress and mint sauce (page 283)
crispy green salad (page 248)

- Mix together the lamb mince, herbs, carrot, spring onions and garlic in a large bowl.
- Add the egg and mix thoroughly.
- Divide evenly into 6–8 portions, roll into a ball then flatten gently.
- Chill in the fridge for 1–2 hours.
- Char-grill (or barbecue) to taste, and serve with watercress and mint sauce and crispy green salad.

CARBOHYDRATE CONTENT PER SERVING: 7 GRAMS

Baked Trout with Pine Nut and Almond Butter

There are many recipes combining trout with almonds – a very successful combination – but add some pine nut and almond butter to fresh trout and you're reaching new heights of gastronomic delight. Vitamin E from almonds and pine nuts will mop up all of your free radicals!

For 2

2 medium trout, cleaned
3 tbsp groundnut oil
75 grams mangetout
75 grams broccoli florets

Pine nut and almond butter

75 grams unsalted butter
50 grams ground pine nuts
50 grams ground almonds
1 tbsp freshly squeezed lemon juice
pinch of rock salt
freshly ground black pepper

- Melt the butter in a small saucepan, stir in the ground pine nuts, almonds and lemon juice and season to taste.
- Place the cleaned trout in a shallow oven-safe baking dish, spoon most of the nut butter inside the trout (as in stuffing), and brush the surface of the trout with the remainder.
- Cover with pierced aluminium foil and bake in the centre of a pre-heated oven at 180°C (gas 4) for 15–20 minutes.

Just before the trout is ready

- Lightly steam the mangetout and broccoli.
- Transfer the baked trout to warm plates and serve immediately with mangetout and broccoli.

CARBOHYDRATE CONTENT PER SERVING: 5 GRAMS

Tiger Prawns with Coconut Milk

Tiger prawns have an aesthetically pleasing appearance, which is an important aspect of any recipe; it doesn't matter how nutritious the meal, if it doesn't look good, it won't be successful. Ask any child! The delicate texture of prawns absorbs the many flavours in this recipe: the sweetness of coconut milk, the hot Tabasco, and the aromatic sweet basil.

For 2

2 tbsp extra-virgin olive oil
1 medium red onion, peeled and sliced
1 garlic clove, peeled and chopped finely
8–10 cooked tiger prawns, shelled and deveined
1 medium red pepper, deseeded and sliced finely
1 medium yellow pepper, deseeded and sliced finely
1 tbsp chopped fresh Thai sweet basil
100 ml light coconut milk
2–3 drops of Tabasco sauce (optional)
pinch of rock salt
freshly ground black pepper
green salad with herbs (page 252)

- Heat the virgin olive oil in a wok and gently sauté the onion and garlic for 1–2 minutes.
- Add the prawns, peppers, and basil, and stir-fry for 2–3 minutes.
- Stir in the coconut milk, add the Tabasco sauce (if desired), and season to taste.
- Simmer gently for 4–5 minutes.
- Serve immediately with green salad with herbs.

CARBOHYDRATE CONTENT PER SERVING: 9 GRAMS
(INCLUDING SALAD)

Spicy Chicken Drumsticks

This is a simple recipe for spicing up chicken drumsticks. It's very quick to prepare and very healthy. The addition of a tasty marinade, which can be easily prepared from stock ingredients in the larder transforms this from a simple to a delicious – and nutritious – meal.

Sesame has been used in cooking since the time of the ancient Egyptians, who may not have known of its value as a rich source of omega-6 essential fatty acids. Then again, maybe they did!

For 2

6 chicken drumsticks, skin on, scored diagonally on each side
2 tbsp extra-virgin olive oil
julienne strips of green chilli, to garnish
coriander vegetables and crème fraîche (page 248)

Marinade

2 tbsp light soy sauce
2 tbsp sweet sherry
1 garlic clove, peeled and chopped finely
2 slices of fresh ginger root, peeled and chopped finely
1 tsp sesame oil

- Mix the soy sauce, sherry, garlic, ginger and sesame oil in a medium bowl, add the drumsticks and marinate for 3–4 hours.
- Brush the drumsticks with extra-virgin olive oil, and barbecue (or grill) for about 10–12 minutes, turning regularly and basting with the marinade.

At the same time

- Prepare the coriander vegetables and crème fraîche.
- When ready, serve the spicy chicken drumsticks with coriander vegetables and crème fraîche, garnished with strips of green chilli.

CARBOHYDRATE CONTENT PER SERVING: 18 GRAMS (3 GRAMS WITHOUT CORIANDER VEGETABLES AND CRÈME FRAÎCHE)

Cream Eggs with Tarragon and Chives

Tarragon is an ancient remedy for toothache, as well as snakebite! Useful in case of unforeseen emergencies.

For 2

20 grams of unsalted butter, divided into 2 cubes
2 large free-range eggs
2 tbsp double cream
2 tsp chopped fresh tarragon
2 tsp chopped fresh chives
freshly ground black pepper
chopped chives, to garnish

- Fill a medium saucepan with warm water to a depth of about 1 cm, bring to the boil, then reduce the heat and stand 2 cocottes in the water for 1–2 minutes to heat through.
- Place a small cube of butter in the base of each cocotte.
- When the butter has melted, gently break an egg into each cocotte.
- Cover, and gently simmer for about 2 minutes.
- Mix the cream with the tarragon and chives, season with freshly ground black pepper, and spoon a tbsp of the cream mixture over each egg.
- Cover, and leave to cook in the gently simmering water for 2 minutes, then serve immediately, garnished with chopped chives.

CARBOHYDRATE CONTENT PER SERVING: 1 GRAM

Turkey and Avocado

In sandwiches or toast, always try to use wholemeal bread, rather than white or brown. Wholemeal bread is rich in vitamin B, and actually slows the digestive process, which is an essential part of healthy nutrition as it allows our body to absorb the nutrients from the food.

For 2

1 medium Hass avocado, halved, stoned, peeled and
  chopped finely
1 tbsp mayonnaise, commercial or home-made
  (page 274)
2 tsp freshly squeezed lemon juice
3 spring onions, chopped into 3–4 cm lengths
$1/2$ tbsp chopped fresh basil
freshly ground black pepper
2 slices of buttered wholemeal toast (optional)
4 slices of cooked turkey breast
4 semi-dried tomatoes with herbs (page 254) or
  commercial sun-dried tomatoes
rocket and olive salad (page 247)

- Mix together the avocado, mayonnaise, lemon juice,
  spring onions, basil and black pepper in a small
  bowl.
- Place two slices of cooked turkey breast on each
  slice of toast (or directly onto the centre of the plate,
  if you don't want an open sandwich).
- Spoon on the avocado mixture, and top with semi-
  dried tomatoes.
- Garnish with sprigs of fresh basil.
- Serve with rocket and olive salad.

CARBOHYDRATE CONTENT PER SERVING: 26 GRAMS
(OR 9 GRAMS WITHOUT BREAD)

Parmesan Salmon

This could also be named 'the vitamin D recipe', as
both salmon and cheese are a rich source of this
vitamin.

For 2

15 grams unsalted butter
15 grams plain flour

150 ml full-cream milk
200 gram tin of red salmon, flaked and bones
   removed
2 tbsp freshly grated Parmesan cheese
2 tbsp freshly grated breadcrumbs
1 tbsp chopped fresh basil
pinch of rock salt
freshly ground black pepper
fresh basil leaves, to garnish

- Melt the butter in a medium saucepan, remove from the heat and stir in the flour.
- Return to a low heat and gradually blend in the milk.
- When the sauce begins to thicken, stir in 1 tbsp of Parmesan cheese and continue to stir constantly until the cheese melts, then stir in the salmon, 1 tbsp of breadcrumbs, and the chopped basil.
- Transfer the mixture to a grill-safe dish, top with a tbsp of Parmesan cheese and a tbsp of breadcrumbs, and grill under a pre-heated moderate grill (no closer than 8 cm from the grill) until the cheese begins to brown.
- Serve immediately, garnished with fresh basil leaves.

CARBOHYDRATE CONTENT PER SERVING: 21 GRAMS

Chapter 4

Sunday Lunch

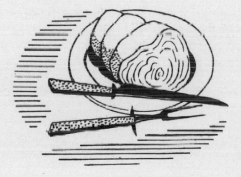

Roast Beef with Mangetout 87
Chicken Marsala 88
Roast Pork with Apple Sauce 90
Tarragon Chicken 90
Beef Pot Roast with Herbs 92
Chicken with Creamy Curry Mayonnaise 93
Roast Lamb with Mint Sauce 94
Roast Chicken with Broccoli 95

Traditional Sunday lunch is often considered a 'heavy' meal, to be avoided on a diet. This is nonsense! With relatively small modifications to Sunday lunch, almost all of the traditional menus can be included in this diet successfully: roast beef with gravy, roast pork with apple sauce, roast lamb with mint sauce, roast turkey . . . The list is virtually endless, and there is virtually no restriction on the quantities. Simply replace the high-carbohydrate elements of the meal (such as potatoes) with vegetables of a lower carbohydrate content and, of course, omit the very-high-carbohydrate Yorkshire pudding (for which there is no low-carbohydrate equivalent, I'm afraid), and the traditional Sunday lunch is back on the agenda for serious dieters. And you can enjoy delicious sauces (described in Chapter 8) to complete the perfect meal. There are few meals less appetising (or edible) than the typical low-calorie diet with no sauces and tasteless dressings!

It really is this simple to lose weight and be healthy.

Roast Beef with Mangetout

Mangetout is a rich source of both vitamins A and C.

For 6

Joint of beef (sirloin, silverside, fore rib or
    topside), approximately 2 kg, preferably on the
    bone (definitely better flavour than boneless)
500 grams mangetout
500 grams carrots, julienne
12 small yellow squash
3 spring onions, chopped finely

- Place the joint (tied with string) in a roasting tin then cook in the centre of a pre-heated oven at 180°C (gas 4) for the following times, depending on how well-cooked you prefer: for beef cooked rare, 20 minutes per 450 grams plus 20 minutes extra; for beef cooked medium, 25 minutes per 450 grams plus 25 minutes extra; for beef well-done, 30 minutes per 450 grams plus 30 minutes extra. Of course, ovens vary, and you may find your oven takes a slightly longer or shorter time to achieve the desired result. Anyone who gives exact instructions for oven cooking has never cooked!
- Shortly before the beef is ready, lightly steam the mangetout, carrots and yellow squash.
- Carve the beef according to the preferred thickness, and serve with either horseradish sauce (page 282), gravy (page 284), or mustard.

CARBOHYDRATE CONTENT PER SERVING: 11 GRAMS
(13 GRAMS WITH HORSERADISH SAUCE, 15 GRAMS WITH GRAVY, AND 12 GRAMS WITH MUSTARD)

Chicken Marsala

This recipe uses baked chicken (rather than fried chicken, which is often quoted for this recipe) as the tender baked chicken fillets will absorb the flavours much more effectively.

For 2

2 chicken breasts, about 150–175 grams each
25 grams of butter, cubed
1 tbsp extra-virgin olive oil
1 garlic clove, peeled and chopped finely
100 ml chicken stock
3 tbsp Marsala
2 tbsp single cream

pinch of rock salt
freshly ground black pepper
2 tsp chopped fresh flat-leaf parsley, to garnish
75 grams of broccoli florets
75 grams of sugarsnap peas

- Place the chicken fillets in a medium baking dish and dot with cubes of butter.
- Cover with pierced aluminium foil, and cook in the centre of a pre-heated oven at 180°C (gas 5) for 35–40 minutes.
- Remove from the oven, cover and set aside.
- Heat the extra-virgin olive oil in a small frying pan and gently sauté the garlic for 1–2 minutes.
- Stir in the stock and Marsala, bring to the boil, then reduce the heat and simmer until the mixture has reduced by about half to two-thirds of the original volume.

At the same time

- Lightly steam the broccoli and sugarsnap peas.
- When the stock mixture has reduced by about half to two-thirds, stir in the cream, season to taste, and heat through gently.
- Pour the sauce over the chicken and garnish with chopped fresh flat-leaf parsley.
- Serve with the lightly steamed broccoli and sugar snap peas.

CARBOHYDRATE CONTENT PER SERVING: 5 GRAMS

Roast Pork with Apple Sauce

Virtually unlimited roast pork on a diet? Highly
nutritious, and you will continue to lose weight at the
safest healthy rate.

For 4

1½ kilogram joint of pork (preferably on the bone)
apple sauce (page 285)
200 grams broccoli florets
2 large red peppers and 2 large yellow peppers, char-
grilled, peeled and sliced thinly (page 239)

- Place the pork joint in a roasting tin and cook in the
centre of a pre-heated oven at 180°C (gas 4) for 30
minutes per 450 grams plus 30 minutes extra
(2 hours 10 minutes for a 1½ kg joint of pork).
- While the pork is cooking, prepare the apple sauce.
- About 10 minutes before the joint is ready, lightly
steam the broccoli and char-grill the peppers.
- When the peppers are cooked, remove the skins,
slice finely and mix the red and yellow peppers
together.
- Carve the pork joint to the desired thickness and
serve with apple sauce, broccoli florets and the
colourful (and highly nutritious) char-grilled peppers.

CARBOHYDRATE CONTENT PER SERVING: 14 GRAMS
(ONLY 4 GRAMS WITHOUT THE APPLE SAUCE!)

Tarragon Chicken

Wine imparts a delicious 'body' to the juices and,
remember, it is not alcoholic! Alcohol boils at a lower
temperature than water, so the alcohol evaporates, and
the flavour remains.

For 2

300 grams skinless chicken breast fillet, sliced thinly
25 grams plain flour
pinch of rock salt
freshly ground black pepper
3 tbsp extra-virgin olive oil
1 large red onion, peeled and sliced finely
1 garlic clove, peeled and chopped finely
1 red pepper, deseeded and sliced finely
100 ml Chardonnay
1 tbsp chopped fresh tarragon
1 tsp chopped fresh flat-leaf parsley
1 tsp Dijon mustard
100 ml single cream
100 grams sugarsnap peas

- Coat the chicken strips in seasoned flour.
- Heat 2 tbsp of virgin olive oil in a medium frying pan and sauté the onion and garlic for 1–2 minutes.
- Add the chicken and cook for 3–4 minutes, stirring frequently.
- Stir in the pepper, Chardonnay, tarragon, flat-leaf parsley and mustard, and simmer very gently for 8–10 minutes.

At the same time

- Lightly steam the sugarsnap peas.
- Stir the single cream into the chicken, and heat through gently.
- Serve immediately with lightly steamed sugarsnap peas.

CARBOHYDRATE CONTENT PER SERVING: 20 GRAMS

Beef Pot Roast with Herbs

Parsnips have the dubious honour of being replaced by potatoes as the major starchy vegetable in our diet.

For 4

1 kilogram joint of beef
2 tbsp plain flour
pinch of rock salt
freshly ground black pepper
4 tbsp extra-virgin olive oil
1 large onion, peeled and sliced
1 garlic clove, peeled and chopped finely
2 carrots, peeled and chopped on the diagonal
1 parsnip, peeled and chopped
50 grams button mushrooms, trimmed, wiped and
   halved
2 bay leaves
250 ml beef stock
1 tbsp chopped fresh basil
1 tbsp chopped fresh rosemary
2 tsp chopped fresh coriander
1 tsp cornflour
2 tbsp water
fresh basil leaves, to garnish

- Coat the meat with seasoned flour.
- Heat 3 tbsp extra-virgin olive oil in a large pan, and brown the meat.
- Remove the joint from the pan, cover and set aside.
- Add 1 tbsp extra-virgin olive oil to the pan, and gently sauté the onion and garlic for 2–3 minutes.
- Add the carrots, parsnip and mushrooms, and stir-fry for 2–3 minutes, then return the meat to the pan, add the bay leaves, basil, rosemary and coriander, and sufficient stock to just cover the vegetables.
- Season to taste, cover, and simmer gently for 1½ hours, turning the meat occasionally.

- Transfer the meat to a serving platter, remove the vegetables with a perforated spoon, and arrange the vegetables around the meat.
- Mix the cornflour with the water to form a smooth paste.
- Gradually add the cornflour paste to the pan, stirring constantly.
- Heat through, and serve the gravy over the pot roast.
- Garnish with sprigs of fresh basil.

CARBOHYDRATE CONTENT PER SERVING: 15 GRAMS

Chicken with Creamy Curry Mayonnaise

Curry mayonnaise with coriander is – yet another – perfect accompaniment to chicken. And the chilli provides a good source of chromium in our diet, which is essential for the function of the hormone insulin.

For 2

2 chicken breasts, skin removed
200 ml creamy curry mayonnaise (page 271)
1 tbsp chopped fresh coriander
fresh coriander leaves, to garnish
crispy green salad (page 248)

- Place the chicken fillets in a shallow baking dish, dot with butter cubes, cover, and bake in the centre of a pre-heated oven at 180°C (gas 4) for 35–40 minutes.
- Remove from the oven and allow to cool, then chop into 2–3 cm cubes.
- Mix the chicken with the mayonnaise and chopped coriander, cover and chill in the fridge for 2–3 hours.
- Serve with a crispy green salad, garnished with fresh coriander leaves.

CARBOHYDRATE CONTENT PER SERVING: 3 GRAMS

Roast Lamb with Mint Sauce

Apart from its healthy antioxidant properties, mint provides the perfect accompaniment to roast lamb, not only in flavour, but also as a potent appetite stimulant.

For 4

1¹/₂ kilogram joint of lamb (tied), preferably
   on the bone for extra flavour
mint sauce (page 285)
250 grams French beans
250 grams carrots, julienne
pinch of rock salt
freshly ground black pepper

- Place the lamb joint in a roasting tin and cook in the centre of a pre-heated oven at 180°C (gas 4) for the following times, depending on how well-cooked you prefer: for medium lamb, 25 minutes per 450 grams plus 25 minutes extra (total of 1 hour 50 minutes for 1¹/₂ kg); for well-done lamb, 30 minutes per 450 grams plus 30 minutes extra (2 hours 10 minutes for 1¹/₂ kg), but always remember that ovens vary in temperatures and cooking times, so you really have to get to know your own oven, which only comes with trial and error.
- About 10 minutes before the lamb is ready, lightly steam the French beans and carrots, then serve the lamb with mint sauce and season to taste.

CARBOHYDRATE CONTENT PER SERVING: 10 GRAMS
(INCLUDING MINT SAUCE)

Roast Chicken with Broccoli

As you will have noticed, there is virtually no restriction on 'normal' life in this diet. You can still enjoy roast chicken (or turkey, pork, lamb, beef), with gravy, for Sunday lunch – or any other time – without adversely affecting the diet. Just restrict the carbohydrates, especially refined carbohydrates, and you will lose weight easily and stay healthy.

For 4

1½ kilogram oven-ready fresh (or thoroughly thawed frozen) chicken, giblets removed
2 tbsp extra-virgin olive oil
gravy (page 284)
200 grams broccoli florets
12 yellow squash

- Wash the chicken, and pat dry.
- Brush the chicken lightly with extra-virgin olive oil.
- Place it in a roasting tin, and cook in the centre of a pre-heated oven at 180°C (gas 4) for 20 minutes per 450 grams plus an extra 20 minutes (i.e. about 1½ hours for a 1½ kg chicken).
- Transfer the chicken to a carving dish, and allow to cool for 5–10 minutes before carving.
- While the chicken is standing, prepare the gravy and lightly steam the broccoli and squash. Serve the carved chicken with the vegetables and gravy.

CARBOHYDRATE CONTENT PER SERVING: < 1 GRAM
(WITHOUT GRAVY), 5 GRAMS (WITH GRAVY)

Chapter 5

Dinner

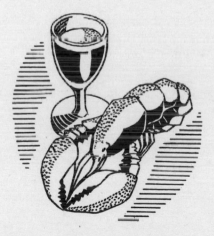

The term 'dinner' includes a wide variety of potential meals, from light supper to formal dinner parties. Obviously, there are significant overlaps between the chapters in this book; many of the recipes in the 'light lunch' and 'quick-and-easy' chapters are equally applicable to dinner in certain circumstances, and vice versa. However the most important aspect is that a nutritionally balanced, low-carbohydrate diet can be adapted to every situation, allowing safe and healthy weight loss combined with improved nutritional well-being.

Sesame Trout with Ginger

This recipe provides omega-6 essential fatty acids from sesame seeds combined with the healthy properties of ginger – which have been recognized for over 2000 years. Ginger helps prevent blood clots, improves circulation, reduces nausea and assists digestion. And there are all the essential amino acids from the trout.

For 2

2 large trout fillets
half a small red pepper, deseeded and sliced finely
3 spring onions, chopped into thin strips,
    approximately 4–5 cm in length
freshly ground black pepper
100 ml full-cream milk
fresh dill and strips of red chilli, to garnish
75 grams of mangetout

Marinade

> 2 tbsp light soy sauce
> 2 tbsp dry sherry
> 2 tsp sesame oil
> 1 garlic clove, peeled and chopped finely
> 2 slices of fresh ginger root, peeled and chopped finely
> pinch of salt

- Mix together the ingredients of the marinade, and set aside.
- Place the trout fillets in the base of a deep oven-safe dish, and pour over the marinade.
- Marinate the trout for 2–3 hours.
- Place the pepper and spring onions on the fish, season to taste, and pour the milk around the fish.
- Cover with pierced aluminium foil, and cook in the centre of a pre-heated oven at 180°C (gas 4) for 12–15 minutes.

At the same time

- Lightly steam the mangetout for 3–4 minutes.
- Serve the sesame trout, garnished with fresh dill and thin slices of red chilli, with lightly steamed mangetout.

CARBOHYDRATE CONTENT PER SERVING: 6 GRAMS

Chilli Tiger Prawns

We have mentioned on several occasions that there are numerous combinations of foods in nature which are gastronomically and nutritionally perfect. Chilli and prawns are another example. We first enjoyed the exquisite pleasure of chilli tiger prawns on a visit to Singapore many years ago. It is a unique flavour which lingers in the memory forever.

Although it is well-known that chilli is a marvellous source of vitamin A and vitamin C, perhaps of less general knowledge is that it has been used for centuries to prevent blood clotting.

For 2

10 cooked tiger prawns, peeled
spinach with chilli and pine nuts (page 242)
lime wedges
lime zest, to garnish

Marinade

1 garlic clove, peeled and grated
1 small red chilli, deseeded and chopped very finely
2 slices of fresh ginger root, peeled and chopped
    finely
2 tbsp light soy sauce
2 tbsp sweet sherry
2 tbsp extra-virgin olive oil
juice of half a lemon, freshly squeezed
1 tsp sesame oil
freshly ground black pepper

- Mix together the ingredients of the marinade in a moderate-sized bowl.
- Shell the tiger prawns. The easiest way to shell a prawn is to remove the head and tail, break off the legs and the shell will then peel easily. Be careful to remove all of the shell; it has an awful texture!
- Marinate the prawns for 3–4 hours.
- Prepare the spinach with chilli and pine nuts.
- Grill or barbecue the prawns for 2–3 minutes, turning once and basting with the marinade.
- Serve the chilli tiger prawns with spinach, chilli, pine nuts and lime wedges, garnished with lime zest.

CARBOHYDRATE CONTENT PER SERVING: 7 GRAMS

Tandoori Pork with Rocket

Cardamom (in garam masala) and rocket are both said to have aphrodisiac properties. So this meal may be more 'spicy' than you expect!

For 2

2 slices of fresh ginger root, peeled and
   chopped finely
1 garlic clove, peeled and chopped finely
1 tsp garam masala
2 tsp chopped fresh coriander
1 tsp ground turmeric
$1/2$ tsp paprika
freshly ground black pepper
150 ml natural yoghurt
250 grams lean pork fillet
100 grams wild rocket, washed
lime wedges
fresh coriander leaves, to garnish

- Mix together the ginger, garlic, garam masala, coriander, turmeric, paprika and pepper in a bowl.
- Stir the mixture into the yoghurt.
- Coat the pork fillets with the spicy yoghurt, then marinate for 4–6 hours in the fridge.
- Place a sheet of aluminium foil on the grill tray, brush lightly with extra-virgin olive oil, and lay the pork fillets on the tray.
- Grill under a high heat, about 8 cm from the grill, for 10–12 minutes, turning once.
- Serve with lime wedges on a bed of wild rocket, garnished with fresh coriander leaves.

CARBOHYDRATE CONTENT PER SERVING: 5 GRAMS

Trout with Watercress and Mint Sauce

The high concentration of antioxidants in watercress,
mint and lime juice make this an incredibly healthy
meal, which also happens to taste delicious.

For 2

8 baby leeks, trimmed and sliced lengthways
2 tbsp extra-virgin olive oil
2 trout fillets
pinch of rock salt
freshly ground black pepper
watercress and mint sauce (page 283)
lime wedges
fresh dill, to garnish

* Lightly steam the leeks.
* Brush the trout fillets with extra-virgin olive oil and
  cook under a medium grill (no closer than 8 cm
  from the grill) for 12–15 minutes, turning once.
* At the same time, prepare the watercress and mint
  sauce.
* Place the trout on a bed of leeks, pour over the
  watercress and mint sauce and garnish with fresh
  dill.
* Serve with lime wedges.

CARBOHYDRATE CONTENT PER SERVING: 5 GRAMS

Spicy Turkey Kebabs

For some unknown reason, roast turkey seems to be
inextricably linked with Yuletide – and no other time of
year. In fact, nothing could be further from the truth.
Turkey can now be bought in the same way as chicken,
either as whole breast fillets (or ready sliced breast) or
drumsticks. As with all pure foods, turkey has a unique

taste and texture, and the ability to absorb appropriate flavours. In this recipe, the delicate aroma of the spices blends with the tangy lemon, and is tempered by the cooling influence of the yoghurt.

For 2

2 skinless turkey breast fillets
    (approximately 150 grams each), cubed
crispy green salad (page 248)
cucumber raita (page 281)

Marinade

2 tsp ground cumin
1 tsp ground coriander
2 tsp garam masala
$1/2$ tsp ground ginger
1 garlic clove, peeled and grated
1 tbsp freshly squeezed lemon juice
125 ml natural yoghurt

- Grate the garlic with a ginger- or garlic-grater.
- Prepare the marinade and marinate the turkey for 4–6 hours in the fridge.
- Remember to soak the wooden skewers during this period, or they will burn when you grill later.
- Thread the skewers with the marinated turkey cubes, and cook under a medium grill, no closer than 8 cm from the grill, for about 8–10 minutes, turning frequently.
- Serve immediately with a crispy green salad and cucumber raita.

CARBOHYDRATE CONTENT PER SERVING: 11 GRAMS (INCLUDING SALAD AND RAITA)

Beef with Chilli

Chilli powder has 100 times the vitamin A content of bananas!

For 2

3 tbsp extra-virgin olive oil
1 medium onion, peeled and sliced
1 garlic clove, peeled and chopped finely
400 grams of stewing steak, cubed
2 tsp hot chilli powder (adjust to individual taste)
1 tbsp tomato purée
200 ml beef stock
pinch of rock salt
freshly ground black pepper
1 large red pepper, deseeded and chopped
red lettuce salad (page 254)

- Heat the extra-virgin olive oil in a large frying pan, brown the beef and sauté the onion and garlic for 3–4 minutes.
- Add the chilli powder, and sauté for a further minute, then stir in the tomato purée and beef stock.
- Season to taste.
- Bring to the boil, then lower the heat and simmer very gently for $1\frac{1}{2}$ hours.
- Add the pepper, and simmer gently for a further $\frac{1}{2}$ hour, then serve with red lettuce salad.

CARBOHYDRATE CONTENT PER SERVING: 19 GRAMS
(INCLUDING 11 GRAMS FOR SALAD)

Calamari and Ginger

Calamari has all the essential amino acids we need to manufacture all of our own body proteins, and many of the vitamins – but not vitamin C. Red and yellow peppers are among the highest sources of vitamin C of all vegetables. And the calamari absorbs the complementary flavours in this recipe to provide the perfect result in every aspect: taste, texture, nutrition and visual delight.

For 2

2 tbsp extra-virgin olive oil
1 tsp sesame oil
75 grams spring onions, chopped (on the diagonal) into 3–4 cm lengths
1 garlic clove, peeled and chopped finely
3 slices of fresh ginger root, peeled and chopped finely
1 small red pepper, deseeded and sliced
1 small yellow pepper, deseeded and sliced
8 large tiger prawns, peeled and deveined
100 grams fresh calamari tubes, sliced into rings
1 tbsp light soy sauce
1 tbsp dry sherry
2 tsp freshly squeezed lemon juice
freshly ground black pepper
100 grams mangetout
1 bok choy, halved

- Heat the extra-virgin olive oil and sesame oil in a wok, and sauté the spring onions and garlic for about a minute.
- Add the ginger, peppers, prawns and calamari, and stir-fry for 3–4 minutes.
- Stir in the soy sauce, sherry and lemon juice, season to taste, and cook for a final 1–2 minutes.

At the same time

- Lightly steam the mangetout and bok choy.

CARBOHYDRATE CONTENT PER SERVING: 6 GRAMS

Shish Kebab

This recipe provides essential amino acids from lamb, vitamin A from tomatoes and red pepper, vitamin C from red and green peppers, and vitamin B_2 from mushrooms. And it tastes delicious!

For 2

250 grams lean lamb, chopped into 2–3 cm cubes
6 cherry tomatoes
1 medium red pepper, deseeded and chopped into
    2–3 cm cubes
1 medium green pepper, deseeded and chopped into
    2–3 cm cubes
12 button mushrooms, wiped
freshly ground black pepper
2 tbsp extra-virgin olive oil
6 wooden skewers, soaked in water for 2–3 hours
    before use
red lettuce salad (page 254)

Marinade

2 tbsp light soy sauce
2 tbsp sweet sherry
1 slice of fresh ginger root, peeled and chopped
    finely
1 garlic clove, grated
1 tsp freshly squeezed lime juice
pinch of rock salt
freshly ground black pepper

- Grate the garlic with a ginger- or garlic-grater.
- Mix together the marinade, and marinate the lamb for 4–6 hours.
- Thread the cubed lamb, tomatoes, peppers and mushrooms on the skewers alternately.
- Season to taste, pour the remaining marinade over the kebabs, and brush with extra-virgin olive oil.
- Grill, or barbecue, on high for 6–8 minutes, turning frequently.
- Serve with red lettuce salad.

CARBOHYDRATE CONTENT PER SERVING: 21 GRAMS
(INCLUDING SALAD)

Honey-glazed Pork

How simple can it be to produce a delicious meal, which is both highly nutritious and cooks in less than 15 minutes? Mustard and honey are a delightful combination, complemented by the addition of a smooth, dry white wine.

For 2

2 lean pork fillets (approx 150 grams each)
lime zest, to garnish
red lettuce salad (page 254)

Marinade

1 tbsp Dijon mustard
1 tbsp clear honey
1 tbsp dry white wine
pinch of cayenne pepper
pinch of rock salt

- Mix together the ingredients of the marinade thoroughly, and coat the pork fillets.

- Marinate the pork in the fridge for 3–4 hours, then place under a hot grill, about 8 cm from the heat, and cook for 10 minutes, turning 3–4 times.
- Garnish with lime zest, and serve with red lettuce salad.

CARBOHYDRATE CONTENT PER SERVING: 23 GRAMS

Trout with Mustard Cream Sauce

A light and nutritious meal which is perfect for either lunch or supper, this dish can be very quickly prepared if the trout is cooked in the microwave oven; in fact, the trout cook to perfection in only 2–3 minutes using this method, which proves that *real fast* food is healthy!

For 2

2 large trout fillets
freshly ground black pepper
100 ml full-cream milk
30 grams butter
2 shallots, peeled and sliced
1 garlic clove, peeled and chopped finely
4 tbsp dry white wine
2 tsp Dijon mustard
100 ml single cream
1 tsp chopped fresh coriander
1 bok choy, halved lengthways

- Place the trout fillets in the base of a baking dish, season to taste, and pour the milk around the fish
- Cover with pierced aluminium foil, and cook in the centre of a pre-heated oven at 180°C (gas 4) for 12–15 minutes.

Or

- Place the trout fillets in a single layer in the base of a microwave-safe dish.
- Microwave on 'high' for two minutes.
- Allow to stand for 1–2 minutes.

At the same time

- Heat the butter in a medium saucepan and sauté the shallots and garlic for 1–2 minutes.
- Add the wine and reduce for 3–4 minutes.
- Add the mustard, cream and coriander and stir constantly for 1–2 minutes over low heat.
- Lightly steam the bok choy for 5–6 minutes.
- Remove the trout from the oven (or microwave), transfer to warm plates with a perforated spoon, and pour over the mustard cream sauce.
- Garnish with fresh coriander leaves, and serve with lightly steamed bok choy.

CARBOHYDRATE CONTENT PER SERVING: 4 GRAMS

Lobster with Basil and Chive Sauce

Lobster is a 'rich' meal in every sense of the word – taste and nutrition. But it needn't be expensive. With rich food, like lobster and salmon, you only need small amounts to satisfy the largest appetite.

For 2

2 raw lobster tails
pinch of rock salt
basil and chive sauce (page 273)
100 grams sugarsnap peas
100 grams yellow squash, quartered lengthways
freshly ground black pepper
fresh basil leaves, to garnish

- Add the lobster tails to a saucepan of boiling water, stir in a pinch of rock salt, and cook for 5–6 minutes.
- Remove from the pan with a perforated spoon, allow to cool, then crack open the shell and extract the lobster meat.

At the same time

- Lightly steam the sugarsnap peas and baby squash.
- Prepare the basil and chive sauce.
- Arrange the lobster meat on the side of the plate, pour over the sauce, and season with freshly ground black pepper.
- Garnish with fresh basil leaves, and serve with the lightly steamed sugarsnap peas and baby squash.

CARBOHYDRATE CONTENT PER SERVING: 12 GRAMS

Turkey with Rosemary and Thyme

The aromatic flavours of the herbs merge with the turkey to form a delicious combination and, as rosemary and thyme provide high levels of natural antioxidants, the nutritional content is excellent.

For 2

4 tbsp extra-virgin olive oil
2 skinless turkey breast fillets, approximately
   125–150 grams each
1 large red onion, peeled and chopped
1 large garlic clove, peeled and chopped finely
1 tbsp chopped fresh thyme
1 tbsp chopped fresh rosemary
200 ml medium white wine
freshly ground black pepper
100 grams of mangetout
100 grams of yellow squash
sprigs of fresh rosemary, to garnish

- Heat 3 tbsp of extra-virgin olive oil in a medium frying pan and sauté the turkey breasts until cooked.
- Remove from the pan and cover.
- Heat the remaining virgin olive oil in the pan and sauté the onion and garlic for 2–3 minutes.
- Return the turkey to the pan, stir in the thyme, rosemary and wine, bring to the boil, then lower the heat and simmer very gently for 20–30 minutes.

Just before the turkey is ready

- Lightly steam the mangetout and yellow squash.
- When the turkey is cooked, adjust the seasoning and serve with lightly steamed mangetout and yellow squash, garnished with sprigs of fresh rosemary.

CARBOHYDRATE CONTENT PER SERVING: 6 GRAMS

Lamb with Basil

Herbs have an incredible concentration of antioxidants – over 100 times the quantity in potatoes!

For 2

25 grams plain flour
250 grams of lean lamb fillet, cubed
3 tbsp extra-virgin olive oil
200 grams of baby onions, peeled
1 garlic clove, peeled and chopped finely
400 ml lamb stock
400 gram tin of plum tomatoes, chopped
1 tbsp tomato purée
1 medium red pepper, deseeded and sliced
1 medium yellow pepper, deseeded and sliced
1 tbsp chopped fresh basil
$1/2$ tbsp chopped fresh coriander
juice of a freshly squeezed lemon
pinch of rock salt
freshly ground black pepper

75 grams of broccoli florets
sprigs of fresh rosemary, to garnish

- Lightly coat the lamb cubes in seasoned flour.
- Heat 2 tbsp of extra-virgin olive oil in a large frying pan, and brown the lamb.
- Transfer to a casserole dish with a perforated spoon, and set aside.
- Heat the remaining olive oil in the pan and sauté the onion and garlic for 1–2 minutes.
- Add the stock, tomatoes and tomato purée, bring to the boil, then lower the heat and gently simmer for 4–5 minutes.
- Stir in the peppers, herbs and lemon juice, and season to taste.
- Transfer to the casserole dish and cover.
- Cook in the centre of a low oven at 140°C (gas 1) for 2–2½ hours.
- Serve the casserole with lightly steamed broccoli, and garnish with sprigs of fresh rosemary.

CARBOHYDRATE CONTENT PER SERVING: 27 GRAMS

Chilli Beef Salad

Strange though it may seem, you can actually omit the chilli in this recipe, without losing the taste. So if you don't like spicy flavours, leave out the chilli! It still tastes delicious, and is very healthy and nutritious.

For 2

250 grams of lean beef fillet
150 grams mixed crispy lettuce leaves (curly endive, coral, green oak leaf, and mizuna) and rocket
1 medium Lebanese cucumber, sliced lengthways
fresh coriander leaves, to garnish

Marinade

1 tbsp oyster sauce
1 tbsp sweet sherry
1 tbsp extra-virgin olive oil
2 slices of fresh ginger root, peeled and chopped
    finely
1 garlic clove, peeled and chopped finely
freshly ground black pepper

Dressing

4 tbsp extra-virgin olive oil
1 tbsp chopped fresh basil leaves
1 tbsp white wine vinegar
1 small red chilli, deseeded and chopped (optional)
1 spring onion, chopped finely
1 stalk of lemon grass, outer leaves removed,
    chopped finely
juice of a freshly squeezed lemon
pinch of rock salt
freshly ground black pepper

- Mix together the ingredients of the marinade, and marinate the beef for 4–6 hours.
- Place the beef in a roasting tin, pour over the marinade, and cover.
- Cook in the centre of a pre-heated oven at 200°C (gas 6) for 25–30 minutes.
- Remove from the oven and allow to cool, then slice finely.
- Add the ingredients of the dressing to a blender and process until smooth, then season to taste.
- Place the salad leaves and cucumber on individual plates, top with the beef, and drizzle over the dressing.
- Garnish with fresh coriander leaves.

CARBOHYDRATE CONTENT PER SERVING: 5 GRAMS

Sesame Pork with Mushrooms

Like all meat and fish products, pork provides us with all of the essential amino acids, however, it has the additional attribute of being a particularly rich source of vitamin B_1. And it blends perfectly with sesame, soy and ginger.

For 2

200 grams of lean pork fillet, sliced thinly
1 tbsp sesame seeds
3 tbsp extra-virgin olive oil
1 tbsp sesame oil
3 spring onions, chopped into 3–4 cm lengths
50 grams sugarsnap peas
1 medium red pepper, deseeded and sliced thinly
100 grams button mushrooms, wiped and halved
freshly ground black pepper
lime zest, to garnish

Marinade

2 tbsp sweet sherry
1 tbsp light soy sauce
1 tsp freshly squeezed lime juice
1 garlic clove, peeled and chopped finely
2 slices of fresh ginger root, peeled and chopped finely
1 tsp cornflour

- Mix together the ingredients of the marinade.
- Add the pork, cover and marinate in the fridge for 3–4 hours.
- Dry stir-fry the sesame seeds in a wok for about 1 minute over medium heat.
- Remove from the wok, and set aside.
- Heat 2 tbsp of extra-virgin olive oil in the wok and stir-fry the pork for 3–4 minutes.
- Remove from the wok with a perforated spoon, and set aside.

117

- Heat the remaining virgin olive oil and sesame oil, and stir-fry the spring onions, sugarsnap peas, pepper and mushrooms for 2–3 minutes.
- Return the pork to the wok, stir in the marinade, season to taste, and stir-fry for 2–3 minutes.
- Garnish with lime zest and sesame seeds, and serve immediately.

CARBOHYDRATE CONTENT PER SERVING: 10 GRAMS

Smoked Trout Pâté

Fats in your diet don't necessarily make you fat! In fact, they only cause weight gain when combined with carbohydrates, so include some of the 'good' pure fats (like cheese) in your diet for health: fats slow the digestive process and satisfy hunger, actually encouraging you to eat less! Cheese and cream (in moderation) are definitely beneficial, not harmful.

Horseradish is a rich source of vitamin C and a gastric stimulant. In this recipe, it blends perfectly with the powerful flavour of smoked trout.

For 2

1 smoked trout, flaked and boned
150 grams of Philadelphia cheese
1 tbsp horseradish sauce (page 282)
2 tbsp single cream
1 tbsp chopped fresh basil
2 tsp chopped fresh coriander
pinch of rock salt
freshly ground black pepper
pinch of paprika and fresh basil leaves, to garnish

- Mix together the smoked trout, cheese, horseradish sauce, cream, basil, and coriander, then season to taste.

- Blend until smooth, and chill for 3–4 hours in the fridge.
- Just before serving, garnish with fresh basil leaves and paprika.

CARBOHYDRATE CONTENT PER SERVING: 4 GRAMS

Beef with Ginger

This recipe includes red wine, which has been scientifically proven to lower the risk of heart disease if consumed in moderation (no more than 2 glasses of red wine per day).

For 2

2 tbsp plain flour
½ tsp ground ginger
pinch of rock salt
freshly ground black pepper
400 grams of braising steak, cubed
3 tbsp extra-virgin olive oil
1 medium onion, peeled and sliced
1 garlic clove, peeled and chopped finely
300 ml beef stock
1 medium green chilli, deseeded and chopped finely
3 slices of fresh root ginger, peeled and chopped finely
200 gram tin of chopped plum tomatoes
2 tsp brown sugar
2 tsp Worcestershire sauce
1 bay leaf
100 ml red wine
1 medium red pepper, deseeded and sliced
1 medium yellow pepper, deseeded and sliced
100 ml sour cream
fresh basil leaves, to garnish

- Coat the beef cubes with seasoned flour (including ground ginger).
- Heat the extra-virgin olive oil in a large frying pan and brown the beef, then add the onion and garlic, and sauté for about 2 minutes.
- Transfer to an oven-safe casserole dish.
- Mix together the stock, chilli, ginger, tomatoes, sugar, Worcestershire sauce, bay leaf and red wine, and pour over the beef.
- Cover, and cook in the centre of a pre-heated moderate oven at 160°C (gas 3) for about 1½–2 hours, depending on the oven.
- Add the peppers, season to taste, and cook for a further 20–30 minutes.
- Remove from the oven, remove the bay leaf and stir in the sour cream.
- Serve immediately, garnished with fresh basil.

CARBOHYDRATE CONTENT PER SERVING: 31 GRAMS

Cod Kebabs with Baby Squash

With a little preparation of the marinade in advance, this dish is quick and nutritious – with delicious results! Vitamin A and C in pepper and squash complement the superb nutritional value of cod.

For 2

400 grams cod fillets, chopped into 2–3 cm cubes
2 tbsp extra-virgin olive oil
4 baby onions, peeled
8 yellow squash
8–10 button mushrooms, wiped
1 large red pepper, chopped into 2–3 cm segments
freshly ground black pepper
red lettuce salad (page 254)

Marinade

2 tbsp light soy sauce
1 tbsp sweet sherry
1 slice fresh ginger root, peeled and chopped finely
1 garlic clove, peeled and chopped finely

- Marinate the cod for 2–3 hours.
- At the same time, soak 6 wooden skewers in cold water before use.
- Thread the skewers with alternate cod cubes, onions, squash, button mushrooms and peppers.
- Brush with olive oil and grill under a hot grill, or barbecue, for 5–6 minutes.
- Serve with red lettuce salad.

CARBOHYDRATE CONTENT PER SERVING: 20 GRAMS
(INCLUDING SALAD)

Barbecue Thai Lamb

Lamb has a delicate texture, which absorbs aromatic spices in a deliciously subtle manner.

For 2

2 tsp garam masala
$^1/_2$ tsp ground cumin
$^1/_2$ tsp ground turmeric
1 small onion, peeled and chopped finely
1 garlic clove, peeled and chopped finely
3 slices of fresh ginger root, peeled and chopped finely
2 sticks of lemon grass, outer leaf discarded and chopped finely
1 tbsp chopped fresh coriander
1 tbsp Thai fish sauce
100 ml coconut milk

250 grams of lean lamb fillet, cubed
fresh coriander leaves, to garnish
crispy green salad (page 248)

- Add the garam masala, cumin and turmeric to a medium pan and dry stir-fry for about a minute.
- Transfer the spices to a food processor, add the onion, garlic, ginger, lemon grass, coriander, fish sauce and coconut milk and blend until smooth.
- Pour the marinade over the lamb, and marinate in the fridge for 3–4 hours.
- Soak the wooden skewers in water.
- Thread the lamb onto the skewers, and barbecue (or grill) for 6–8 minutes, turning frequently.
- Garnish with fresh coriander leaves, and serve immediately with a crispy green salad.

CARBOHYDRATE CONTENT PER SERVING: 4 GRAMS

Beef Casserole with Cabernet Sauvignon

Studies have shown that red wine (in moderation) is definitely beneficial for your health, probably due to the presence of the antioxidant 'resveratrol'.

For 2

2 tbsp extra-virgin olive oil
400 grams lean blade or topside steak, cubed
1 medium red onion, peeled and diced
1 tbsp plain flour
2 medium garlic cloves, peeled and chopped finely
100 ml Cabernet Sauvignon
200 ml beef stock
12–14 small onions, peeled
100 grams button mushrooms, wiped and halved
1 tbsp chopped fresh basil
$1/2$ tbsp chopped fresh coriander

freshly ground black pepper
75 grams of broccoli
75 grams of French beans
sprigs of fresh basil, to garnish

- Heat the extra-virgin olive oil in a wok and brown the steak cubes.
- Add the onion and garlic, and sauté for 2–3 minutes, then remove from the heat and stir in the flour.
- Stir in the red wine and beef stock, and simmer for 3–4 minutes, stirring frequently.
- Pour into a casserole dish, cover and bake in the centre of a pre-heated oven at 160°C (gas 3) for 1½–2 hours.
- Add the onions and bake for a further 15 minutes, then add the mushrooms, basil and coriander.
- Season to taste, and return to the oven for a further 10–12 minutes.
- Garnish with sprigs of fresh basil, and serve with lightly steamed broccoli and French beans.

CARBOHYDRATE CONTENT PER SERVING: 22 GRAMS

Chicken Cacciatore

There are many variations on the standard recipe, all of which are nutritionally superb, with essential amino acids from chicken, antioxidants from garlic, tomatoes and herbs, and vitamin B from mushrooms.

For 4

4 tbsp extra-virgin olive oil
8 chicken drumsticks, with skin
1 large onion, peeled and diced
1 garlic clove, peeled and chopped finely
400 gram tin of chopped plum tomatoes
1 tbsp tomato purée

100 ml chicken stock
100 ml dry white wine
1 tbsp chopped fresh oregano
1 tbsp chopped fresh basil
100 grams of black olives
100 grams of button mushrooms, wiped and halved
freshly ground black pepper
fresh oregano leaves, to garnish
green salad with herbs (page 252)

- Heat 2 tbsp of extra-virgin olive oil in a large saucepan and brown the chicken drumsticks.
- Remove from the pan with a perforated spoon, set aside and cover.
- Heat the remaining virgin olive oil, and sauté the onion and garlic for 2–3 minutes.
- Stir in the tomatoes, tomato purée, chicken stock, white wine, herbs, olives and mushrooms, and season to taste.
- Bring to the boil, then lower the heat and simmer for about 10 minutes.
- Return the chicken to the pan and gently simmer for a further 40–45 minutes.
- Garnish with fresh oregano leaves, and serve with green salad with herbs.

CARBOHYDRATE CONTENT PER SERVING: 14 GRAMS
(INCLUDING SALAD)

Citrus Cod and Rocket

Cod is a rich source of all essential amino acids and many essential nutrients, but not vitamin C, which is amply provided by both oranges and limes. The sweetness of the orange juice combines with the sharpness of lemon and lime juice to produce a natural sweet-and-sour sauce, which blends admirably with the texture of the cod.

For 2

300 grams of cod fillet, chopped into 3–4 cm cubes
100 grams of rocket
lemon wedges

Marinade

juice of half a freshly squeezed orange
juice of half a freshly squeezed lime
1 tbsp sweet sherry
2 tbsp extra-virgin olive oil
1 slice of fresh ginger root, peeled and chopped
   finely
1 tsp chopped fresh mint
freshly ground black pepper

- Prepare the marinade.
- Marinate the cod for 4–6 hours in the fridge.

At the same time

- Soak the wooden skewers in water for before use.
- Thread the cod onto the skewers, and cook under a hot grill (or barbecue) for 6–8 minutes, turning and basting with the marinade frequently.
- Serve on a bed of fresh rocket, with lemon wedges.

CARBOHYDRATE CONTENT PER SERVING: 4 GRAMS

Lamb with Basil Sour Cream

Here you'll find vitamin A from rosemary, vitamin C from lemon, and members of the B group of vitamins from lamb. Nature seems to combine health and flavour perfectly.

For 2

300 grams lean lamb fillet, cubed
chopped fresh chives and sprigs of rosemary, to garnish
green salad with herbs (page 252)

Marinade

3 tbsp extra-virgin olive oil
1 tbsp sweet sherry
1 garlic clove, peeled and grated finely
2 sprigs of fresh rosemary
2 tsp freshly squeezed lemon juice
pinch of rock salt
freshly ground black pepper

Basil sour cream

150 ml sour cream
1 tbsp chopped fresh basil
2 tsp chopped fresh chives

- Grate the garlic with a ginger- or garlic-grater.
- Marinate the lamb for 4–6 hours in the fridge. Soak the wooden skewers for 2–3 hours before use.

At the same time

- Mix together the sour cream, basil and chives, cover and cool in the fridge.
- Thread the meat onto the skewers and cook under a hot grill for 6–8 minutes, turning frequently.
- Pour the basil sour cream over the lamb skewers, garnish with chopped chives and fresh sprigs of rosemary, and serve with green salad with herbs.

CARBOHYDRATE CONTENT PER SERVING: 6 GRAMS

Spicy Thai Swordfish

Swordfish is 100% essential proteins, and the ingredients in this recipe are complementary in both taste and nutrition, from the vitamin C in the lemon juice to the vitamin A in the lemon grass!

For 2

2 swordfish steaks (about 150–175 grams each)
2 tsp sesame seeds
1 bok choy, halved lengthways

Marinade

1 tbsp Thai fish sauce
1 tbsp sweet sherry
juice of a freshly squeezed lemon
1 large garlic clove, peeled and chopped finely
3 slices of fresh ginger root, peeled and chopped
   finely
1 green chilli, deseeded and chopped finely
1 stick of lemon grass, outer leaves removed and
   chopped finely
1 tbsp chopped fresh coriander
1 tbsp chopped fresh Thai sweet basil

- Mix together the ingredients of the marinade.
- Marinate the swordfish steaks for about 1 hour, turning once.
- Dry stir-fry the sesame seeds for about a minute.
- Steam the marinated swordfish for 5–6 minutes.

At the same time

- Lightly steam the bok choy for 3–4 minutes.
- Serve the swordfish steaks with lightly steamed bok choy, and garnish with lightly toasted sesame seeds.

CARBOHYDRATE CONTENT PER SERVING: 4 GRAMS

Beef Curry with Yoghurt

Chillis are believed to improve the circulation, stimulate digestion (not much doubt there), clear respiratory congestion, and even increase the rate we burn calories. Their effects are definitely cooled by soothing yoghurt.

For 2

4 tbsp extra-virgin olive oil
300 grams lean beef fillet, cubed
1 medium onion, peeled and sliced
1 garlic clove, peeled and chopped finely
$1/2$ small green chilli, deseeded and chopped finely (optional)
2 slices of fresh ginger root, peeled and chopped finely
1 tsp ground cumin
1 tsp ground cardamom
100 ml beef stock
1 tbsp dry sherry
50 ml single cream
50 ml natural yoghurt
freshly ground black pepper
julienne strips of red chilli, to garnish

- Heat 2 tbsp of extra-virgin olive oil in a wok and brown the beef, then remove from the wok with a perforated spoon and cover.
- Heat the remaining olive oil in the wok and sauté the onion for 2–3 minutes, then add the garlic, chilli, ginger, cumin and cardamom, and cook over a low heat for 2–3 minutes, stirring frequently.
- Return the beef to the wok, stir in the stock and sherry, cover and simmer gently for about an hour.
- Stir in the yoghurt and cream, season to taste, and gently heat through the mixture, then serve immediately, garnished with julienne strips of red chilli.

CARBOHYDRATE CONTENT PER SERVING: 6 GRAMS

Cod with Chive and Parsley Butter Sauce

Herb butter sauce is absorbed to perfection by the delicate texture of white fish, producing a delicious gastronomic combination. Chives and parsley complement the flavour of fish perfectly, and also provide healthy antioxidant protection from vitamin C.

For 2

2 cod fillets, approximately 150 grams each
25 grams butter, cubed
100 ml full-cream milk
freshly ground black pepper
caper and olive salad (page 253)

Chive and parsley butter sauce

3 tbsp dry white wine
2 tsp freshly squeezed lemon juice
1 tsp freshly squeezed lime juice
1 tbsp double cream
50 grams butter
1 tbsp chopped fresh chives
2 tsp chopped fresh flat-leaf parsley
freshly ground black pepper
flat-leaf parsley leaves, to garnish

- Place the cod fillets in a shallow oven-safe dish and pour the milk around the fish.
- Season with freshly ground black pepper, and dot with butter.
- Cover, and cook in the centre of a pre-heated oven at 180°C (gas 4) for 15 minutes. Remove with a perforated spoon and serve on warm plates.

At the same time

- Add the wine, lemon juice and lime juice to a small

saucepan, bring to the boil, reduce by about half, and stir in the cream.

- Remove from the heat and add the butter.
- Return to a low heat, and gently melt the butter, stirring constantly.
- Stir in the chives and flat-leaf parsley and season to taste.
- Pour the herb butter sauce over the cod fillets and garnish with flat-leaf parsley.
- Serve with caper and olive salad.

CARBOHYDRATE CONTENT PER SERVING: 10 GRAMS
(INCLUDING SALAD)

Turkey Curry with Almonds

Turkey is particularly suitable for curries as it retains its texture and flavour throughout the prolonged slow-cooking process. Almonds add a piquant taste – and are a particularly rich source of calcium (surprisingly), potassium and vitamin E.

For 2

4 tbsp extra-virgin olive oil
1 medium onion, peeled and sliced
3 slices of fresh ginger root, peeled and chopped finely
1 garlic clove, peeled and chopped finely
$1/2$ small red chilli, deseeded and chopped finely
1 tsp ground turmeric
1 tsp ground cumin
1 tsp ground coriander
150 ml chicken stock
400 gram tin of chopped plum tomatoes
250–300 grams of turkey breast fillet, sliced thickly on the diagonal

1 small red pepper, deseeded and sliced
1 small yellow pepper, deseeded and sliced
1 tbsp chopped fresh chives
1 tbsp chopped fresh coriander
50 grams slivered almonds
freshly ground black pepper
fresh coriander leaves and almonds (chopped into
    thin slivers), to garnish

- Heat 2 tbsp extra-virgin olive oil in a large frying pan and sear the turkey for 2–3 minutes.
- Remove from the pan with a perforated spoon, and set aside.
- Heat the remaining extra-virgin olive oil in the pan and sauté the onion for 2–3 minutes.
- Add the ginger, garlic, chilli, turmeric, cumin and ground coriander, and stir-fry over a gentle heat for 1–2 minutes.
- Stir in the stock and tomatoes, bring to the boil, then lower the heat and gently simmer for 6–8 minutes.
- Return the turkey to the pan and gently simmer for 20 minutes.
- Add the peppers and simmer for a further 15 minutes.
- Stir in the chives, coriander and almonds (reserving a few for garnish), season to taste, and simmer for a final 5 minutes before serving.
- Garnish with fresh coriander leaves and slivers of chopped almonds.

CARBOHYDRATE CONTENT PER SERVING: 14 GRAMS

Spicy Haddock with Stir-fried Vegetables

The combination of essential amino acids and vitamins from haddock, antioxidants from herbs, and omega-6 essential fatty acid from sesame oil tastes simply delicious!

For 2

200 grams of haddock fillets, boned and flaked
1 tbsp chopped fresh basil
2 shallots, peeled and diced finely
1 rasher of bacon, diced finely
1 tbsp light soy sauce
3–4 drops of Tabasco sauce
freshly ground black pepper
1 egg white
2 tbsp extra-virgin olive oil
1 garlic clove, peeled and chopped finely
2 spring onions, chopped into 3–4 cm lengths
75 grams mangetout
1 small green pepper, deseeded and chopped finely

Sauce

2 tbsp light soy sauce
2 tbsp sweet sherry
1 tsp sesame oil
½ tsp cornflour

- Mix together the haddock, basil, shallots, bacon, soy sauce, Tabasco sauce and egg white in a bowl, season to taste, and form into small ball shapes.
- Steam the fish balls for about 10–12 minutes, until well-cooked.

At the same time

- Mix together the ingredients of the sauce in a small bowl.

- Heat the olive oil in a wok and stir-fry the garlic, spring onions, mangetout and pepper for 2–3 minutes, add the sauce, and season to taste.
- Cook for a further 2 minutes and serve with the haddock fish balls.

CARBOHYDRATE CONTENT PER SERVING: 7 GRAMS

Chilli Prawn Soufflé

Once again, the delightful combination of chillis and prawns, this time in a soufflé, which adds a completely new dimension to the combination. Chillis were originally brought to Europe by Christopher Columbus. Their health-giving antioxidant properties are matched only by their unique flavour, and the zest they impart to every recipe.

For 2

2 tbsp extra-virgin olive oil
1 garlic clove, peeled and chopped finely
1 small red chilli, deseeded and chopped finely
100 grams cooked prawns, shelled and deveined
3 large free-range eggs, separated
25 grams butter
25 grams plain flour
150 ml full-cream milk
1 tbsp chopped fresh coriander
pinch of rock salt
freshly ground black pepper
finely chopped spring onion, to garnish

- Heat the virgin olive oil in a medium saucepan and sauté the garlic and chilli for 1–2 minutes.
- Stir in the prawns, and cook over medium heat for about 2 minutes.

133

- Separate the eggs, beat the yolks, and whisk the whites until firm.
- Melt the butter in a small saucepan, then gradually beat in the flour and milk, stirring constantly until the mixture is evenly thickened.
- Remove from the heat and allow to cool for 2–3 minutes, stirring occasionally.
- Beat in the egg yolks, stir in the prawn mixture and coriander, and season to taste.
- Beat in a tbsp of egg white to the mixture, then gradually 'fold' the egg whites into the mixture.
- Lightly butter a soufflé dish, gently spoon in the mixture evenly, and bake in the centre of a pre-heated oven at 190°C (gas 5) for 25–30 minutes. Ovens vary; the deciding factor is whether the soufflé has risen.
- Garnish with finely chopped spring onion, and serve immediately.

CARBOHYDRATE CONTENT PER SERVING: 19 GRAMS

Chicken Paprika

Paprika (like chilli) is another member of the capsicum (or pepper) family. It has an immensely high vitamin A content, and is therefore very rich in powerful antioxidants – which remove free radicals and keep us healthy!

For 2

2 chicken breasts, about 150 grams each
50 grams butter, cubed
2 tbsp extra-virgin olive oil
1 medium onion, peeled and diced
1 garlic clove, peeled and chopped finely
1 tbsp plain flour

1 tbsp paprika
100 ml chicken stock
3 large plum tomatoes, peeled and diced
2 tsp tomato purée
100 grams button mushrooms, wiped and halved
   lengthways
200 ml sour cream
freshly ground black pepper
75 grams mangetout
sprigs of fresh tarragon, to garnish

- Place the chicken fillets in a shallow baking dish, dot with butter cubes, and bake in the centre of a pre-heated oven at 180°C (gas 4) for 35–40 minutes.
- Remove from the oven and allow to cool, then slice into thin strips.
- Heat the extra-virgin olive oil in a medium frying pan and sauté the onion and garlic for 1–2 minutes.
- Add the chicken to the pan, and stir in the flour and paprika.
- Stir in the stock, tomatoes and tomato purée, season to taste, and simmer for 10 minutes.
- Add the mushrooms and simmer for a further 5 minutes.

At the same time

- Lightly steam the mangetout.
- Stir in the sour cream to the chicken paprika in the pan, and heat through gently for a further minute.
- Serve immediately with lightly steamed mangetout, garnished with sprigs of fresh tarragon.

CARBOHYDRATE CONTENT PER SERVING: 20 GRAMS

Beef Stroganoff

Quercertin is one of the strongest antioxidants known, and the most common source of this health-giving chemical is . . . onions!

For 2

3 tbsp extra-virgin olive oil
250 grams lean steak (preferably rump or fillet), sliced thinly
1 medium red onion, peeled and sliced
1 garlic clove, peeled and chopped finely
$\frac{1}{2}$ tsp ground paprika
100 grams button mushrooms, wiped and halved
150 ml beef stock
I tbsp tomato purée
pinch of rock salt
freshly ground black pepper
100 ml sour cream
75 grams broccoli florets
chopped fresh chives and fresh parsley leaves, to garnish

- Heat 2 tbsp extra-virgin olive oil in a frying pan and brown the steak.
- Remove from the pan with a perforated spoon, cover and set aside.
- Heat the remaining olive oil in the pan and gently sauté the onion, garlic, paprika and mushrooms for 2–3 minutes. Stir in the beef stock and tomato purée, return the steak to the pan, and season to taste.
- Bring to the boil, reduce the heat and simmer gently for 10–15 minutes, stirring occasionally.
- Remove from the heat, stir in the sour cream, and serve immediately.
- Garnish with chopped fresh chives and fresh parsley leaves, and serve with lightly steamed broccoli.

CARBOHYDRATE CONTENT PER SERVING: 6 GRAMS

Pork Curry

Hot, spicy and healthy, or it can just be spicy and healthy if you leave out the chilli! Curry doesn't have to be hot to taste delicious.

For 2

4 tbsp extra-virgin olive oil
350 grams lean pork, chopped into 3–4 cm cubes
1 medium onion, peeled and sliced
2 garlic cloves, peeled and chopped finely
1 green chilli, deseeded and chopped finely
    (substitute a small red chilli if you prefer a hot
    curry)
2 slices of fresh ginger root, peeled and chopped
    finely
1 tsp ground turmeric
1 tsp ground coriander
1 tsp ground cumin
3 large plum tomatoes, peeled and chopped
1 tbsp tomato purée
100 ml pork stock
50 ml dry white wine
1 tbsp chopped fresh coriander
pinch of rock salt
freshly ground black pepper
1 tbsp chopped fresh chives, to garnish

- Heat 2 tbsp extra-virgin olive oil in a wok and brown the pork.
- Remove from the wok with a perforated spoon, set aside and cover.
- Heat the remaining virgin olive oil in the wok and sauté the onion and garlic for 2–3 minutes.
- Add the chilli, ginger, turmeric, ground coriander and cumin and cook over low heat for 2–3 minutes.
- Stir in the tomatoes, tomato purée, stock and wine.

- Return the pork to the pan, cover and gently simmer for about 1 hour.
- Stir in the fresh coriander, season to taste and simmer for a final 10 minutes.
- Just before serving, garnish with chopped chives.

CARBOHYDRATE CONTENT PER SERVING: 10 GRAMS

Salmon Steaks with Herbs

This dish combines the superbly nutritious qualities of salmon with the antioxidants in herbs. Incidentally, tarragon can also be used to treat snakebite – according to the ancient Romans!

For 2

2 tbsp extra-virgin olive oil
2 salmon steaks, approximately 150–175 grams each
pinch of rock salt
freshly ground black pepper
1 tbsp chopped fresh tarragon
1 tbsp chopped fresh chives
1 tbsp freshly squeezed lemon juice
lemon wedges
sprigs of fresh tarragon, to garnish
char-grilled vegetables with sesame seeds (page 229)

- Place the salmon steaks on individual sheets of aluminium foil, and brush with extra-virgin olive oil.
- Season to taste and sprinkle the herbs evenly over the salmon.
- Close the foil parcels and cook in the centre of a pre-heated oven at 180°C (gas 4) for about 20 minutes, depending on the oven.
- Remove the salmon from the parcels, drizzle over freshly squeezed lemon juice and garnish with sprigs of fresh tarragon.

- Serve immediately with lemon wedges and chargrilled vegetables with sesame seeds.

CARBOHYDRATE CONTENT PER SERVING: 26 GRAMS

(1 GRAM WITHOUT VEGETABLES)

Honey and Ginger Chicken

The flavour of chicken blends perfectly with the sweetness of the honey and the spicy ginger. And both peppers and chilli are members of the capsicum family, which is well-known to be an excellent source of the antioxidant vitamins A and C. Once again, it simply proves that healthy food tastes delicious, if prepared correctly.

For 2

2 chicken breast fillets, sliced into thin strips
3 tbsp extra-virgin olive oil
1 red onion, peeled and sliced vertically into wedges
1 medium yellow pepper, deseeded and chopped into
    large cubes
1 medium red pepper, deseeded and chopped into
    large cubes
1 tbsp chopped fresh basil
freshly ground black pepper
fresh basil leaves, to garnish

Marinade

2 slices of fresh ginger root, peeled and finely
    chopped
1 green chilli, deseeded and chopped finely
1 garlic clove, peeled and chopped finely
2 tbsp light soy sauce
2 tbsp sweet sherry
1 tbsp clear honey
juice of half a lemon, freshly squeezed

- Mix together the ingredients of the marinade, and marinate the chicken strips for 3–4 hours.
- Heat 2 tbsp of extra-virgin olive oil in the wok, and stir-fry the onion and peppers for 2–3 minutes.
- Remove from the wok with a perforated spoon and set aside.
- Heat the remaining virgin olive oil in the wok, and stir-fry the chicken strips for 2–3 minutes.
- Add the remaining marinade and stir-fry for another minute.
- Return the vegetables to the wok, add the basil and season to taste.
- Stir-fry for 1 final minute before serving, garnished with fresh basil leaves.

CARBOHYDRATE CONTENT PER SERVING: 19 GRAMS

Lamb Casserole

Casserole cooking retains all of the healthy nutrients, allowing the various complementary flavours to blend together.

For 4

50 grams unsalted butter
600 grams lamb neck fillet, cubed
1 large red onion, peeled and sliced
1 garlic clove, peeled and chopped finely
1 parsnip, peeled and chopped
1 large carrot, peeled and chopped
75 grams of French beans
100 grams of button mushrooms, wiped and halved
25 grams of plain flour
250 ml lamb stock
400 gram tin of chopped plum tomatoes
1 tbsp chopped fresh rosemary
1 tbsp chopped fresh flat-leaf parsley

pinch of rock salt
freshly ground black pepper

- Melt the butter in a medium saucepan and brown the lamb cubes, then remove from the pan with a perforated spoon and transfer to an oven-safe casserole dish.
- Sauté the onion and garlic for 1–2 minutes, then add the parsnip, carrot, French beans and mushrooms, and cook for a further 2–3 minutes.
- Stir in the flour, then blend in the stock, tomatoes, rosemary and parsley, and season to taste.
- Cook over medium heat for 2–3 minutes, then transfer to the casserole dish.
- Cover and cook in the centre of a pre-heated oven at 160°C (gas 2) for 1½–2 hours, depending on the oven.

CARBOHYDRATE CONTENT PER SERVING: 16 GRAMS

Salmon and Basil Pâté

The king of herbs with the king of fish. The term 'basil' is derived from the Greek word for 'king', which is most appropriate for such a nutritious and versatile herb. Apart from its undoubted gastronomic uses, basil has also been used as a mild tranquillizer for centuries. You can use fresh or tinned salmon. The tinned variety has similar nutritional qualities as fresh salmon; it still has excellent flavour, but not quite as good as its fresh counterpart.

For 2

400 grams of salmon fillet (or 440 gram tin of red
    salmon, drained, and bones removed)
100 ml full-cream milk
25 grams butter

2 shallots, peeled and chopped finely
1 garlic clove, peeled and chopped finely
1 tbsp freshly squeezed lemon juice
2 tbsp Chardonnay
1 tbsp chopped fresh basil
1 tsp chopped fresh coriander
2 tbsp freshly grated breadcrumbs (one <u>small</u> slice of
   toasted bread – brown or white)
2 egg whites
50 grams melted butter
freshly ground black pepper
sprigs of fresh coriander, to garnish

- Place the salmon fillet in a baking dish and pour the milk around the salmon.
- Cover with pierced aluminium foil, and cook in the centre of a pre-heated oven at 180°C (gas 4) for about 20 minutes.
- Remove from the oven and set aside to cool.

Or instead you could

- Replace the above with 440 grams of tinned red salmon, drained and bones removed.
- Heat 25 grams of butter in a small saucepan and sauté the shallots and garlic for 2–3 minutes.
- Flake the salmon in a medium mixing bowl, add the shallots, garlic, lemon juice, Chardonnay, basil, coriander, breadcrumbs, separated egg whites and melted butter.
- Season to taste, and mix thoroughly.
- Line a loaf tin with aluminium foil and press the pâté mixture firmly in the base of the tin.
- Close the foil parcel loosely, and cook in the centre of a pre-heated oven at 180°C (gas 4) for 40–45 minutes.
- Remove and set aside to cool before serving.

CARBOHYDRATE CONTENT PER SERVING: 16 GRAMS

Lamb with Mustard Cream Sauce

Cream slows the digestion, which is essential for an effective diet, allowing the body to absorb all of the essential nutrition from the food.

For 2

4 tbsp extra-virgin olive oil
250 grams lean lamb fillet, cubed
1 medium red onion, peeled and sliced
1 garlic clove, peeled and chopped finely
60 ml Chardonnay
1 tbsp chopped fresh coriander
freshly ground black pepper
100 ml single cream
1 tbsp wholegrain mustard
75 grams of sugarsnap peas
75 grams of carrot, julienne
fresh coriander leaves, to garnish

- Heat 2 tbsp of extra-virgin olive oil in a medium frying pan and brown the lamb, then reduce the heat and cook the lamb for a further 6–8 minutes, stirring frequently.
- Remove from the pan with a perforated spoon, and set aside.
- Heat the remaining oil in the pan and sauté the onion and garlic for 1–2 minutes.
- Add the Chardonnay and simmer to reduce by about half.
- Return the lamb to the pan, stir in the coriander, season to taste, and simmer for 3–4 minutes.
- Stir in the mustard and cream over low heat, and gently heat through.
- Garnish with fresh coriander leaves, and serve immediately with lightly steamed sugar snap peas and julienne carrots.

CARBOHYDRATE CONTENT PER SERVING: 9 GRAMS

Spicy Tiger Prawns with Coconut

Prawns have a marvellous ability to absorb spicy flavours, producing a delectable mixture of taste, texture and nutrition.

For 2

2 tsp ground cumin
1 tsp ground turmeric
2 tsp ground coriander
2 tbsp extra-virgin olive oil
1 medium onion, peeled and sliced
1 garlic clove, peeled and chopped finely
1 medium green chilli, deseeded and chopped finely
10 cooked tiger prawns, heads and shells removed
1 tbsp chopped fresh coriander
100 ml coconut cream
freshly ground black pepper
75 grams sugarsnap peas
1 large yellow pepper, deseeded and sliced finely
fresh coriander leaves, to garnish

- Dry stir-fry the cumin, turmeric and ground coriander over medium heat for about 1 minute.
- Add the extra-virgin olive oil and sauté the onion, garlic and chilli for 2 minutes, stirring frequently.
- Add the tiger prawns and stir-fry for about 2 minutes.
- Stir in the coconut cream and coriander, season to taste and heat through gently for 1–2 minutes.

At the same time

- Lightly steam the sugarsnap peas and pepper.
- Serve the spicy tiger prawns with the sugarsnap peas and pepper, garnished with fresh coriander leaves.

CARBOHYDRATE CONTENT PER SERVING: 14 GRAMS

Chicken with Macadamia Nuts

Having lived in Australia for many years – where macadamias grow prolifically – we know how versatile these nuts are: in Queensland, they are incorporated into foods as diverse as chocolate and butter! The distinctive qualities of macadamias complement the contrasting flavours and nutritional content of chicken and ginger.

For 2

2 tbsp extra-virgin olive oil
300 grams skinless chicken breast, sliced finely
50 grams unsalted butter
1 medium brown onion, peeled and sliced
1 garlic clove, peeled and chopped finely
75 grams button mushrooms, wiped and halved
2 slices fresh root ginger, peeled and chopped finely
1 tbsp plain flour
200 ml full-cream milk
pinch of rock salt
freshly ground black pepper
50 grams macadamia nuts
100 grams broccoli florets

- Heat the extra-virgin olive oil in a medium frying pan and cook the chicken strips over moderate heat for 3–4 minutes, stirring frequently.
- Remove the chicken from the pan with a perforated spoon and set aside.
- Melt the butter and sauté the onion and garlic for 1–2 minutes.
- Add the mushrooms and ginger and cook for 1–2 minutes.
- Remove from the heat and stir in the flour.
- Return to a low heat and gradually blend in the milk.

- Return the chicken to the mixture and season to taste. Simmer over a low heat for 4–5 minutes.

At the same time

- Lightly steam the broccoli.
- Stir the macadamia nuts into the chicken mixture.
- Heat through gently then serve immediately with lightly steamed broccoli.

CARBOHYDRATE CONTENT PER SERVING: 9 GRAMS

Chilli Prawns with Coriander

All members of the onion family are healthy, and shallots are no exception, but you have to be careful in a low-carbohydrate diet as they have a higher carbohydrate content. In general, the smaller the size of shallot, the stronger the flavour.

For 2

10–12 tiger prawns, pre-cooked
2 tbsp extra-virgin olive oil
2 shallots, peeled and diced
1 garlic clove, peeled and chopped finely
1 medium green chilli, deseeded and chopped finely (optional)
2 tsp freshly squeezed lemon juice
1 tbsp chopped fresh coriander
1 tbsp chopped fresh chives
1 tbsp crème fraîche
freshly ground black pepper
150 grams wild rocket

- Shell and devein the pre-cooked tiger prawns, and set aside.
- Heat the virgin olive oil in a medium frying pan and sauté the shallots, garlic and chilli for 1–2 minutes.

- Stir in the lemon juice, coriander and chives, add the tiger prawns and cook over low heat for 2–3 minutes.
- Remove from the heat and set aside to cool.
- Stir in the crème fraîche and season to taste.
- Serve on a bed of wild rocket leaves.

CARBOHYDRATE CONTENT PER SERVING: 7 GRAMS

Teriyaki Salmon

One of the delightful aspects of this diet is that you can include alcohol, without worrying about calories, because alcohol will only cause weight gain if combined with sugars. The salmon absorbs the Teriyaki sauce to merge beautifully with the unique flavour of fennel. Of course, the nutritional benefits of potassium from fennel and vitamin C from mangetout are an added bonus of this incredibly healthy recipe.

For 2

2 salmon steaks, approximately 150–175 grams
    each, and no more than 2 cm thick
100 grams mangetout
1 fennel bulb, peeled and halved

Teriyaki sauce

2 tbsp saké (Japanese rice wine)
2 tbsp mirin (Japanese sweet wine)
2 tbsp Japanese soy sauce (shoyu) (Chinese soy
    sauce is too strong!)
$1/2$ garlic clove, peeled and grated

- Mix together the ingredients of the Teriyaki sauce.
- Place the salmon steaks in a shallow baking dish and pour over the Teriyaki sauce.

- Cover, and marinate for 3–4 hours, basting several times.
- Grill the salmon under a hot grill for 4–5 minutes per side, turning once.

As the salmon is cooking

- Lightly steam the fennel and mangetout.
- Serve the Teriyaki salmon with lightly steamed mangetout and fennel.

CARBOHYDRATE CONTENT PER SERVING: 11 GRAMS

Spicy Pork with Asparagus

Very little preparation, and ready in minutes. Almost as fast as 'fast food', and infinitely healthier.

For 2

250 grams lean pork fillet, sliced finely
30 grams plain flour
pinch of rock salt
$1/2$ tsp turmeric
$1/2$ tsp chilli powder
$1/2$ tsp ground coriander
2 tbsp extra-virgin olive oil
1 medium red onion, peeled and chopped
1 garlic clove, peeled and chopped finely
100 grams of fresh asparagus
25 grams of cashew nuts, chopped

- Mix together the flour, salt, turmeric, chilli powder and coriander, then coat the pork strips in the seasoned flour.
- Heat the virgin olive oil in a medium frying pan and cook the pork, stirring frequently, for about 3–4 minutes.

- Add the onion and garlic, and cook for a further 2 minutes.
- Add the cashew nuts and heat through for about 2 minutes, stirring frequently.
- As the pork is cooking, lightly steam the asparagus, and serve immediately.

CARBOHYDRATE CONTENT PER SERVING: 20 GRAMS

Chicken and Mushroom Casserole

Prepare in advance, and enjoy later. This is a deliciously healthy meal, which still has only the same amount of carbohydrate, per serve, as a single slice of bread!

For 4

4 large skinless chicken portions,
    approximately 300 grams each
30 grams unsalted butter
1 large red onion, peeled and sliced
1 garlic clove, peeled and chopped finely
30 grams plain flour
400 ml chicken stock
pinch of rock salt
freshly ground black pepper
1 bay leaf
1 tbsp chopped fresh basil
2 tsp chopped fresh coriander
150 grams button mushrooms, wiped and halved
thin strips of red and green chilli, to garnish
    (optional)

- Heat half the butter in a medium frying pan and brown the chicken.
- Transfer the chicken to a deep oven-safe casserole dish.

- Melt the remaining butter in the pan, add the onion and garlic to the pan, and sauté for 1–2 minutes.
- Remove the pan from the heat and stir in the flour.
- Return to a low heat and gradually stir in the stock until the sauce begins to thicken.
- Add the bay leaf, season to taste, and transfer to the casserole dish.
- Cover, and cook in the centre of a pre-heated oven at 180°C (gas 4) for 30–35 minutes.
- Stir in the basil, coriander and mushrooms, and return to the oven for another 20–25 minutes.
- Serve immediately, garnished with strips of fresh red and green chilli (optional).

CARBOHYDRATE CONTENT PER SERVING: 17 GRAMS

Chilli Lamb Kebabs

Chillies have twice the vitamin C content of lemons or limes!

For 2

350 grams of lean lamb, cubed
julienne strips of red chilli and fresh coriander
    leaves, to garnish

Marinade

1 large green chilli, deseeded and chopped finely (or a small red chilli if your taste is hot!)
2 slices of fresh ginger root, peeled and chopped finely
1 garlic clove, peeled and chopped finely
1 tbsp clear honey
1 tbsp light soy sauce
1 tbsp chopped fresh coriander

2 tsp freshly squeezed lime juice
1 tbsp sweet sherry
pinch of rock salt
freshly ground black pepper

- Mix together the chilli, ginger, garlic, honey, soy sauce, coriander, lime juice and sherry, season to taste and marinate the lamb for 2–4 hours in the fridge.

At the same time

- Soak the wooden skewers in water.
- Thread the lamb on the skewers, and grill under a medium grill (no closer than 8–10 cm from the grill) for about 10 minutes, turning frequently.
- Serve with crispy green salad, garnished with julienne strips of red chilli and fresh coriander leaves.

CARBOHYDRATE CONTENT PER SERVING: 13 GRAMS
(INCLUDING SALAD)

Crab with Herbs

This is a delightful variation of a popular Brazilian entrée, but it can be equally successful as a light lunch or supper dish with caper and olive salad.

For 2

2 tbsp extra-virgin olive oil
1 medium red onion, peeled and diced
1 garlic clove, peeled and chopped finely
1 medium round tomato, peeled and diced
200 grams of white crabmeat, pre-cooked
1 tbsp chopped fresh basil
1 tbsp chopped fresh dill
1 tsp paprika

50 ml light coconut milk
2–3 drops of Tabasco sauce
25 grams of fresh breadcrumbs
small pinch of rock salt
freshly ground black pepper
40 grams of freshly grated Parmesan cheese
caper and olive salad (page 253)

- Heat the virgin olive oil and gently sauté the onion and garlic for 2–3 minutes.
- Stir in the tomato, crabmeat, basil, dill, paprika, coconut milk, Tabasco sauce and breadcrumbs.
- Season to taste, and cook over a low heat for 5–6 minutes.
- Spoon the mixture into 4 scallop shells (or ramekins), top with the Parmesan cheese, and place under a moderate grill, no closer than 8 cm from the grill, until the cheese melts.
- Serve immediately, with caper and olive salad.

CARBOHYDRATE CONTENT PER SERVING: 22 GRAMS
(INCLUDING SALAD), 14 GRAMS (WITHOUT SALAD)

Beef Casserole

Oregano is wild marjoram, and has been used for centuries to relieve rheumatism and reduce fevers. Obviously the early pharmacists recognized its antioxidant properties, long before we knew of the existence of antioxidants.

For 4

750 grams casserole steak, cubed
2 tbsp plain flour
pinch of rock salt
freshly ground black pepper
3 tbsp extra-virgin olive oil

1 large brown onion, peeled and sliced
1 garlic clove, peeled and chopped finely
2 large carrots, peeled and sliced
100 grams of button mushrooms, wiped and halved
400 gram tin of plum tomatoes
400 ml beef stock
1 tbsp chopped fresh oregano (or 1 tsp dried oregano)

- Coat the beef in seasoned flour, then heat the virgin olive oil in a large frying pan and brown the beef.
- Transfer the beef to an oven-safe casserole dish.
- Gently sauté the onion and garlic for 1–2 minutes, then add the carrots and cook for 3–4 minutes.
- Finally, add the mushrooms, and cook for a further minute, then transfer the vegetables to the casserole dish, stir in the tomatoes and stock, season to taste and cook slowly in the centre of a pre-heated oven at 160°C (gas 2) for 1½-2 hours.
- Remove the casserole from the oven, stir in the (preferably fresh) oregano, and return to the oven for a final 15 minutes before serving.

CARBOHYDRATE CONTENT PER SERVING: 14 GRAMS

Whiting in Spicy Batter

Cumin and turmeric have been used to settle gastric complaints for over 5000 years. There certainly won't be any gastric complaints from this recipe!

For 2

1 tsp ground cumin
1 tsp ground turmeric
½ tsp chilli powder (optional)
2 large free-range eggs, beaten
1 small white onion, peeled and grated
1 garlic clove, peeled and grated

2 slices of fresh ginger root, peeled and grated
1 tbsp chopped fresh coriander
2 tsp freshly squeezed lemon juice
pinch of rock salt
freshly ground black pepper
4 medium whiting fillets, approximately 75 grams each
2 tbsp plain flour
4 tbsp extra-virgin olive oil
fresh coriander leaves, to garnish
red lettuce salad (page 254)

- Grate the garlic and ginger with a ginger- or garlic-grater.
- Dry stir-fry the ground cumin, turmeric and chilli powder in a small frying pan over medium heat for about a minute, then set aside to cool.
- Mix together the beaten eggs with the onion, garlic, ginger, spices and lemon juice, and season to taste.
- Coat the fillets with the egg mixture, then dust with flour.
- Heat the extra-virgin olive oil in a medium frying pan and fry the fish for about 2 minutes per side, turning once.
- Garnish with fresh coriander leaves, and serve with red lettuce salad.

CARBOHYDRATE CONTENT PER SERVING: 25 GRAMS
(INCLUDING SALAD)

Creamy Smoked Haddock Pâté

The wonderful diversity of flavours present in cold-water fish provide the adventurous cook with an almost limitless variety of gastronomic combinations. For the nutritionist, it's even easier, because all fish are nutritionally superb. The unique taste of smoked haddock blends marvellously with the smooth cream and hot chilli in this recipe, and chillis, like all members of the capsicum family, are a rich source of the essential antioxidant vitamins A and C.

For 2

150 grams smoked haddock
100 ml full-cream milk
1 bay leaf
25 grams butter
4 tbsp double cream, beaten until just beginning to
    thicken
2 tsp freshly squeezed lemon juice
$1/2$ tsp Worcestershire sauce
3–4 drops Tabasco sauce
$1/2$ green chilli, deseeded and grated fincly (optional)
1 tbsp chopped fresh basil
1 tbsp melted butter
fresh coriander leaves, to garnish

- Place the haddock in the base of an oven-safe dish, pour the milk around the fish and add the bay leaf.
- Cover with pierced aluminium foil, and bake in the centre of a pre-heated oven at 180°C (gas 4) for 10–12 minutes.
- Remove the haddock with a perforated spoon, and allow to cool.
- Flake the haddock, and beat in 25 grams of butter. Blend until smooth.
- Gradually stir the cream into the haddock, adding the lemon juice, Worcestershire sauce, Tabasco sauce, grated chilli (optional), and basil.
- Transfer the mixture to ramekins, and top with clarified butter.
- Chill in the fridge for 1 hour.
- Just before serving, garnish with fresh coriander leaves.

CARBOHYDRATE CONTENT PER SERVING: 6 GRAMS

Liver with Mushrooms

Sage and thyme are rich sources of vitamin A, which is one of the most important antioxidants in our diet.

For 2

3 tbsp extra-virgin olive oil
300 grams lamb's liver
1 medium brown onion, peeled and sliced thinly
1 garlic clove, peeled and chopped finely
100 grams of button mushrooms, trimmed, wiped and halved
1 tbsp chopped fresh sage
1 tbsp chopped fresh thyme
1 tbsp freshly squeezed lemon juice
pinch of rock salt
freshly ground black pepper
75 grams yellow squash
75 grams mangetout
sprigs of fresh thyme, to garnish

- Heat the extra-virgin olive oil in a large frying pan and braise the liver for about a minute on each side.
- Add the onion and garlic, and gently sauté for about 2–3 minutes.
- Stir in the mushrooms, sage, thyme, and lemon juice, season to taste, and gently stir-fry for 5–6 minutes, stirring frequently and turning the liver once.
- Serve immediately with lightly steamed yellow squash and mangetout, garnished with sprigs of fresh thyme.

CARBOHYDRATE CONTENT PER SERVING: 8 GRAMS

Tuna and Oregano Casserole

For some inexplicable reason, fresh tuna is not one of the most popular fish in Europe, yet the tinned variety could not be more popular. Tuna is simply superb nutritionally, whether fresh or tinned, and is one of the best sources of omega-3 essential fatty acids.

For 2

3 tbsp extra-virgin olive oil
250 grams fresh tuna, boned and cubed
1 medium red onion, peeled and diced
1 garlic clove, peeled and chopped finely
1 medium red pepper, deseeded and chopped into large segments
400 gram tin of chopped plum tomatoes
1 tbsp chopped fresh oregano
$1/2$ green chilli, deseeded and chopped finely
75 ml fish stock
pinch of rock salt
freshly ground black pepper
red lettuce salad (page 254)
fresh coriander leaves, to garnish

- Heat 2 tbsp of the extra-virgin olive oil in a frying pan, and sear the tuna for about a minute.
- Remove the tuna from the pan with a perforated spoon, transfer to an oven-safe baking dish and cover.
- Add the remaining tbsp of olive oil to the pan, and sauté the onion, garlic, and pepper for 2–3 minutes.
- Add the tomatoes, oregano, chilli and stock. Season to taste, and simmer for 3–4 minutes.
- Transfer the mixture to the oven-safe baking dish, cover with pierced aluminium foil, and cook in the centre of a pre-heated oven at 190°C (gas 5) for 25–30 minutes.

- Serve with red lettuce salad, and garnish with fresh coriander leaves.

CARBOHYDRATE CONTENT PER SERVING: 22 GRAMS
(INCLUDING SALAD)

Cheese and Chives Soufflé

Cheese and chives are a perfect combination of flavour, texture and nutrition, and the immense variety of cheeses provides an endless variety of different meals and tastes.

For 2

3 large free-range eggs, separated
25 grams butter
25 grams plain flour
150 ml full-cream milk
50 grams Gruyère cheese, grated
25 grams Parmesan cheese, grated
1 tbsp chopped fresh chives
pinch of rock salt
freshly ground black pepper
sprigs of fresh basil, to garnish

- Separate the eggs, beat the yolks, and whisk the whites until firm.
- Melt the butter in a small saucepan, then add the flour and milk, stirring constantly until the mixture thickens.
- Remove from the heat and allow to cool for 2–3 minutes, stirring occasionally.
- Season to taste, then stir in the grated cheese, chives and egg yolks.
- Gradually 'fold' the egg whites into the mixture.
- Lightly butter two individual soufflé dishes, gently spoon in the mixture evenly, and bake in the centre

of a pre-heated oven at 190°C (gas 5) for 25–30 minutes. Ovens vary; the deciding factor is whether the soufflé has risen.

- Serve immediately, garnished with sprigs of fresh basil.

CARBOHYDRATE CONTENT PER SERVING: 25 GRAMS

Swordfish Steaks with Asparagus

This recipe combines two very rich flavours – swordfish and asparagus. Once again, nature combines gastronomic delight with nutritional perfection. Swordfish is a rich source of essential amino acids, and asparagus provides a complementary rich source of potassium and the antioxidant vitamins A, C and E.

For 2

2 medium swordfish steaks, approximately 150–175 grams each
25 grams butter, cubed
50 grams basil pesto sauce (page 276)
100 ml crème fraîche
pinch of rock salt
freshly ground black pepper
small bunch of asparagus, washed and trimmed
lime wedges
fresh coriander leaves, to garnish

- Place the swordfish steaks in an oven-proof baking dish.
- Dot with the butter cubes, cover with pierced aluminium foil, and cook in the centre of a pre-heated oven at 180°C (gas 4) for about 15–20 minutes.

At the same time

- Lightly steam the asparagus.

- Mix the basil pesto sauce with the crème fraîche, heat gently through and season to taste.
- Pour the sauce over the swordfish.
- Garnish with fresh coriander leaves, and serve with lightly steamed asparagus and lime wedges.

CARBOHYDRATE CONTENT PER SERVING: 4 GRAMS

Emmental Aubergine

Aubergines have an immense nutritional value as a source of vitamins B_1, B_2, B_3 and C, which perfectly complements the vitamin D in cheese.

For 4

1 large aubergine
rock salt
4 tbsp extra-virgin olive oil
1 medium red onion, peeled and sliced
1 garlic clove, peeled and chopped finely
400 gram tin of chopped plum tomatoes
1 tbsp tomato purée
2 tsp chopped fresh oregano
1 tbsp chopped fresh basil
freshly ground black pepper
25 grams of Parmesan cheese, freshly grated

Cheese sauce

25 grams plain flour
25 grams butter
200 ml full-cream milk
50 grams Emmental cheese, freshly grated
freshly ground black pepper

- Slice the aubergine into thin slices, place the slices in a colander, sprinkle with salt, and allow to stand for 20–30 minutes, then rinse thoroughly and pat dry.

- Heat 2 tbsp of the extra-virgin olive oil in a medium frying pan and sauté the aubergine slices for 1–2 minutes per side, pat dry, cover and set aside.
- Heat the remaining olive oil, and gently sauté the onion and garlic for 2–3 minutes.
- Stir in the tomatoes, tomato purée, oregano and basil, and season to taste.
- Bring to the boil, and gently simmer for 5 minutes.
- Prepare the white sauce according to the method on page 272, and stir in the Emmental cheese until it has melted.
- Place a layer of aubergine slices in the base of a circular oven-proof dish, top with a sprinkling of cheese sauce, then a layer of tomato and herb sauce.
- Add another layer of aubergine slices, and repeat the process until the ingredients are exhausted.
- Top with a layer of Parmesan cheese, and cook in the centre of a pre-heated oven at 180°C (gas 4) for about 40 minutes.
- Serve immediately, garnished with fresh basil leaves.

CARBOHYDRATE CONTENT PER SERVING: 15 GRAMS

Swordfish with Mustard and Honey

Mustard and honey have both been recognized as potent aphrodisiacs for thousands of years, so be careful with this recipe!

For 2

1 tsp wholegrain mustard
8–10 crushed black peppercorns
1 tbsp clear honey
2 medium swordfish steaks, approximately
    150–175 grams each
25 grams butter, cubed

red lettuce salad (page 254)
fresh coriander leaves, to garnish

- Mix together the mustard, peppercorns and honey.
- Coat the swordfish steaks with the marinade and marinate for 4–6 hours in the fridge.
- Grill the swordfish steaks for 12–14 minutes under a medium grill, turning once.
- Serve with red lettuce salad, garnished with fresh coriander.

CARBOHYDRATE CONTENT PER SERVING: 23 GRAMS
(INCLUDING SALAD)

Smoked Mackerel Pâté

This is a delicious recipe for smoked mackerel pate, which is full of flavour and nutrition. Mackerel is one of the richest sources in our diet of the protective omega-3 essential fatty acids. Combined with the antioxidant vitamin E from the avocado – no more free radicals after this meal!

For 2

200 grams of smoked mackerel, skinned, boned and flaked
1 medium, ripe Hass avocado, halved, peeled, stoned and chopped
50 grams Philadelphia cream cheese
1 tbsp freshly squeezed lemon juice
freshly ground black pepper
fresh coriander leaves, to garnish
caper and olive salad (page 253)

- Add the flaked mackerel, avocado, cream cheese and lemon juice to a food processor.
- Season to taste, and blend until smooth.
- Chill in the fridge for 2–3 hours.

- Just before serving, garnish with fresh coriander leaves, and serve with caper and olive salad.

CARBOHYDRATE CONTENT PER SERVING: 10 GRAMS
(INCLUDING SALAD)

Cheese and Parma Ham Soufflé

Apart from their obvious value as an excellent source of essential amino acids, vitamins and minerals, eggs are also a rich source of the antioxidant mineral selenium.

For 2

3 large free-range eggs, separated
25 grams butter
25 grams plain flour
150 ml full-cream milk
$1/2$ tsp dry mustard
50 grams Parma ham, diced
50 grams mild Cheddar cheese, grated
1 tbsp chopped fresh oregano
pinch of rock salt
freshly ground black pepper

- Separate the eggs, beat the yolks, and whisk the whites until firm.
- Melt the butter in a medium saucepan, remove from the heat and stir in the flour.
- Return to a low heat and gradually blend in the milk.
- Remove from the heat and allow to cool for 2–3 minutes, stirring occasionally.
- Season to taste, then stir in the mustard, ham, grated cheese, oregano and egg yolks.
- Gradually 'fold' the egg whites into the mixture.
- Lightly butter a soufflé dish, gently spoon in the

mixture evenly, and bake in the centre of a pre-heated oven at 190°C (gas 5) for 25–30 minutes. Ovens vary; the deciding factor is whether the soufflé has risen. Serve immediately.

CARBOHYDRATE CONTENT PER SERVING: 13 GRAMS

Taramasalata

Try to be adventurous – particularly with fish. Seafood has a natural variety of different tastes and textures. Providing they are not overcooked (and ruined), you can gently merge different tastes with the natural saltiness of the sea. Smoked cod roe is deliciously complemented, both nutritionally and gastronomically, by chives and green salad.

For 2

1 thin slice of white bread, crust removed
2 tbsp full-cream milk
150 grams smoked cod roe, skin removed
$1/2$ garlic clove, peeled and chopped finely
$1/2$ small brown onion, peeled and grated finely
3 tbsp extra-virgin olive oil
1 tbsp freshly squeezed lemon juice
freshly ground black pepper
chopped fresh chives, to garnish
crispy green salad (page 248)

- Soak the bread in the milk, drain through a sieve, and chop finely.
- Stir in the cod roe, onion and garlic, and mix in the virgin olive oil gradually.
- Add the lemon juice, and season to taste with freshly ground black pepper (salt will probably not be necessary as cod roe is naturally salty).
- Blend until smooth and chill in the fridge for 3–4 hours before serving.

- Just before serving, garnish with chopped fresh chives, and serve with crispy green salad.

CARBOHYDRATE CONTENT PER SERVING: 11 GRAMS
(INCLUDING SALAD)

Beef Korma

This is a delicious variation on the traditional recipe, using beef instead of lamb, and cashew nuts rather than the traditional almonds.

For 2

350 grams of lean beef, cubed
4 tbsp extra-virgin olive oil
$1/2$ medium red onion, peeled and sliced
1 tbsp tomato purée
100 ml beef stock
50 ml natural yoghurt
50 ml single cream
25 grams of raw unsalted cashew nuts
freshly ground black pepper
fresh coriander leaves, to garnish
green salad with herbs (page 252)

Marinade

1 medium red onion, peeled and diced finely
1 garlic clove, peeled and chopped finely
$1/2$ tsp cardamom seeds
1 tsp ground cumin
1 tsp ground coriander
2 slices of fresh ginger root, peeled and chopped finely
pinch of cayenne pepper

- Add the ingredients of the marinade to a mortar, and grind to a paste.
- Brush the beef with 2 tbsp of virgin olive oil.

- Coat the beef with the mixture, and marinate for 2–3 hours.
- Heat the extra-virgin olive oil in a large frying pan, and sauté the onion for 2–3 minutes.
- Add the beef, and cook over a low heat for 7–8 minutes, then stir in the tomato purée and stock.
- Simmer gently for 40–45 minutes, season to taste, and stir in the yoghurt, cream and cashew nuts.
- Heat through gently, garnish with fresh coriander leaves, and serve with green salad with herbs.

CARBOHYDRATE CONTENT PER SERVING: 10 GRAMS

Salmon with Herbs

This is a variation of the traditional recipe for 'gravlax', of which there are many subtle variations on the central theme of fresh salmon with dill. The classic recipe includes sprinkling sugar over the salmon with dill; a teaspoonful can be included if you wish – without significantly affecting a low-carbohydrate diet – but is not really necessary. It is quite difficult to prepare this dish for two, in view of the methods required, so we have given a recipe which serves 4–6.

For 4

2 salmon fillets, approximately 200 grams each
2 tsp rock salt
1 tsp freshly ground white peppercorns
1 tbsp chopped fresh dill
1 tbsp freshly squeezed lemon juice

- Place the fillets in a dish, flesh uppermost, and sprinkle the salt, pepper and fresh dill over the surface of one fillet.
- Lay the other fillet on top (flesh-to-flesh), and wrap in either greaseproof paper or aluminium foil.

- Lay a flat plate (larger than the salmon) on the salmon, place a moderate weight on top, and keep undisturbed in the fridge for two days.
- Unwrap it carefully, drain off any liquid, and slice thinly.
- Roll up the slices, and drizzle over a few drops of lemon juice (to taste).

CARBOHYDRATE CONTENT PER SERVING: < 1 GRAM

Pork Casserole with Oregano

A winter warmer in every sense, and with lycopene in tomatoes and tomato purée, and vitamin C from red pepper, this recipe is certain to mop up any remaining free radicals.

For 2

3 tbsp extra-virgin olive oil
350 grams lean pork fillet, chopped into large cubes
8 baby onions, peeled
1 garlic clove, peeled and chopped finely
1 tbsp plain flour
200 ml pork stock
400 gram tin of chopped plum tomatoes
1 tbsp tomato purée
1 tbsp chopped fresh oregano
100 ml dry white wine
1 medium red pepper, deseeded and sliced
100 grams of button mushrooms, wiped and halved
pinch of rock salt
freshly ground black pepper
fresh basil leaves, to garnish

- Heat 2 tbsp of extra-virgin olive oil in a medium frying pan and brown the pork.
- Transfer the pork to an oven-safe casserole dish with a perforated spoon, and set aside.

- Heat the remaining virgin olive oil and lightly sauté the onions and garlic, then remove from the heat and stir in the flour.
- Add the stock, tomatoes, tomato purée, oregano and wine.
- Season to taste, and gently simmer for 10 minutes.
- Transfer to the casserole dish, cover, and cook in the centre of a pre-heated oven at 160°C (gas 2) for about an hour.
- Add the pepper and mushrooms, and cook for a further 20–25 minutes.
- Just before serving, garnish with fresh basil leaves.

CARBOHYDRATE CONTENT PER SERVING: 23 GRAMS

Tuna and Salmon Sashimi

This dish requires a little preparation time, but no cooking, because it's raw fish, Japanese-style. You either like raw fish or you don't, but it's certainly nutritious!

For 2

150 grams raw tuna fillet, skin removed
150 grams raw salmon, skin removed
wasabi (horseradish – very hot!)
Japanese soy sauce
1 carrot, julienne
3 spring onions, sliced finely on the diagonal

- Chill the fish in the fridge for at least 2–3 hours, then slice the fillets into thin slices.
- A major element of Japanese cooking is presentation, so arrange the slices of tuna and salmon on the plate aesthetically, with wasabi, julienne carrot and spring onions, and a small bowl of Japanese soy sauce (not Chinese soy sauce – too strong).

CARBOHYDRATE CONTENT PER SERVING: 5 GRAMS

Smoked Haddock with Prawns

For some unknown reason, recipes which combine fish
and shellfish are relatively uncommon. The tastes
complement one another perfectly, and the nutrition
cannot be bettered by any other food. Try this
delightful combination of smoked haddock with prawns
and we are sure you will agree.

For 2

25 grams butter
25 grams plain flour
200 ml full-cream milk
2 large smoked haddock fillets (approximately 150
 grams each), bones and skin removed, and
 chopped finely
100 ml double cream
1 garlic clove, peeled and chopped finely
2 large, fresh, free-range eggs, beaten
1 tbsp chopped fresh dill
1 tbsp chopped fresh basil
50 grams frozen prawns, thawed
freshly ground black pepper
50 grams freshly grated Gruyere cheese
150 grams of asparagus

- Melt the butter in a small saucepan, then remove
  from the heat and stir in the flour.
- Return to the heat and gradually add the milk,
  stirring constantly.
- Remove from the heat, once again, and stir in the
  haddock, cream, garlic, eggs, dill, basil and prawns.
- Place in a medium oven-safe baking dish, and season
  to taste with pepper (not salt, as smoked haddock is
  salty).
- Cover with pierced aluminium foil, and cook in the
  centre of a pre-heated oven at 180°C (gas 4) for
  about 20 minutes, depending on the oven.

- Remove from the oven, top with the freshly grated
  Gruyère cheese, and return to the oven for about
  5 minutes.

Just before the haddock and prawns are ready

- Lightly steam the asparagus.
- Transfer the baked smoked haddock and prawns to
  warm plates, and serve with lightly steamed asparagus.

CARBOHYDRATE CONTENT PER SERVING: 17 GRAMS

Cod and Basil Casserole

Casseroles are usually considered the prerogative of
beef, lamb, pork and poultry, but of course seafood add
their own unique flavours and characteristics to
casseroles, and should be included in our diet as much
as possible. Cod is a particularly useful fish for
casseroles, as white fish tend to absorb other flavours –
especially herbs – without the overpowering flavour of
some of the 'richer' oily fish.

For 2

2 cod steaks, approximately 150 grams each, skin
  and bones removed
1½ tbsp plain flour
pinch of rock salt
freshly ground black pepper
2 tbsp extra-virgin olive oil
1 medium red onion, peeled and sliced finely
1 garlic clove, peeled and chopped finely
75 grams button mushrooms, wiped and halved
1 medium yellow pepper, deseeded and sliced thinly
200 gram tin of chopped plum tomatoes
1 tbsp chopped fresh basil
2 tsp chopped fresh coriander
100 grams broccoli florets

- Coat the cod steaks with seasoned flour.
- Heat the virgin olive oil in a small frying pan and sear the cod.
- Transfer the cod to an oven-safe casserole dish.
- Gently sauté the onion and garlic in the frying pan for about a minute, then add the mushrooms and pepper for a further 1–2 minutes.
- Transfer the vegetables to the casserole dish, stir in the tomatoes, basil and coriander, season to taste, and cook in the centre of a pre-heated oven at 180°C (gas 4) for 30–35 minutes.

At the same time

- Lightly steam the broccoli florets.
- Serve the casserole immediately with lightly steamed broccoli florets.

CARBOHYDRATE CONTENT PER SERVING: 18 GRAMS

Stir-fried Chilli Beef

The Szechuan pepper in Chinese five-spice is not a pepper, but rather the berries of a prickly ash tree, and chilli is actually a member of the pepper family. Confused?

For 2

200 grams lean beef fillet, sliced thinly
4 tbsp extra-virgin olive oil
1 tsp sesame oil
3 spring onions, chopped into 3–4 cm lengths
1 garlic clove, peeled and chopped finely
3 slices of fresh ginger root, peeled and chopped fincly
1 green chilli, deseeded and chopped finely
1 medium yellow pepper, deseeded and sliced thinly
1 medium red pepper, deseeded and sliced thinly

75 grams mangetout
75 grams broccoli florets
1 tsp ground Chinese five-spice
50 grams beansprouts
pinch of rock salt
freshly ground black pepper
fresh basil and coriander leaves, to garnish

Marinade

2 tbsp light soy sauce
2 tbsp sweet sherry
1 tsp cornflour
1 garlic clove, peeled and chopped finely

- Mix together the ingredients of the marinade, and marinate the beef strips for 3–4 hours.
- Heat 2 tbsp of extra-virgin olive oil in a wok and stir-fry the beef for about 2 minutes.
- Remove from the wok with a perforated spoon and set aside.
- Heat the remaining olive oil and sesame oil, then sauté the spring onions, garlic, ginger and chilli for 1–2 minutes.
- Add the peppers, mangetout, broccoli and Chinese five-spice, and stir-fry for 2 minutes.
- Return the beef to the wok, add the beansprouts and the remainder of the marinade, season to taste, then stir-fry for a final 2–3 minutes.
- Serve immediately, garnished with fresh basil and coriander leaves.

CARBOHYDRATE CONTENT PER SERVING: 8 GRAMS

Cod with Coriander

Peppers, chilli, tomato, coriander and chives.
Antioxidants in the form of vitamins A and C *par
excellence*. Combined with the essential amino acids in
cod, it is impossible to imagine a more colourful,
delicious and nutritious meal.

For 2

2 shallots, peeled and diced
1 small garlic clove, peeled and chopped finely
1 tbsp tomato purée
4 tbsp tomato juice
1 tbsp chopped fresh coriander
freshly ground black pepper
2 tbsp extra-virgin olive oil
2 large cod fillets, 150–175 grams each, skinned and
   boned
2 tbsp freshly grated Parmesan cheese
chives and pepper salsa (page 257)
fresh coriander leaves, to garnish

- Mix together the diced shallots, garlic, tomato purée,
  tomato juice, coriander and pepper in a medium bowl.
- Brush an oven-safe casserole dish with virgin olive
  oil, then place the cod fillets in the casserole dish.
- Top with the tomato/coriander mixture, sprinkle over
  the grated Parmesan cheese, and cook in the centre
  of a pre-heated oven at 180°C (gas 4) for
  15–20 minutes.

At the same time

- Prepare the chives and pepper salsa.
- Serve the baked cod and coriander with chives and
  pepper salsa, garnished with fresh coriander leaves.

CARBOHYDRATE CONTENT PER SERVING: 10 GRAMS
(INCLUDING THE SALSA)

Chapter 6

Quick-and-Easy Meals

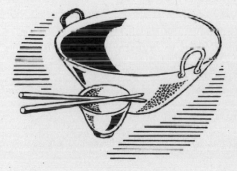

This chapter is the essence of the book. So many of us lead such a hectic pace of life that healthy eating is usually the unfortunate casualty, with inevitable effects on our health in later years. There just doesn't seem to be enough time. This chapter will prove that simply is not the case; healthy, nutritious weight loss can be *easily* achieved with delicious quickly-prepared recipes. Once again, the secret is preparation; place your health on the same level as all of your other priorities, and you will be healthy. And it really doesn't take much time to do this. All you have to do is think about what you intend to eat *in advance*, and make sure you have a supply of the appropriate foods in your kitchen cupboards. The problem for most people is that they pay no attention to the next meal until it's time to eat! This simply won't work, for either your health or your diet. Decide what you intend to prepare for breakfast, lunch or dinner on the evening previously, and the diet works. It will only take a few minutes. Cereals at breakfast, or rice and pasta with the evening meal are favourite foods largely because they are quick to prepare. Prawn fu-yung, beefburgers with herbs, or peppered salmon steaks with lime are equally quick to prepare – and much more nutritious – but they require a little preparation in advance. Not much; all you have to do is decide the types of meals in advance, buy the necessary ingredients when you are shopping, and remember to take them out of the freezer in the morning!

Once again, the secret of successful dieting is simple

preparation and shopping. Decide what you intend to eat in advance, make a shopping list, and buy the necessary ingredients on your next shopping trip. Always keep a store of essential ingredients (see page 5) and you will never be tempted by the inevitable 'quick fix' of the carbohydrate demons: bread, pasta, rice and biscuits. Remember, these foods have virtually no nutritional value. They are high-carbohydrate 'fillers', and unless you happen to be running a marathon (and are able to burn off calories very quickly), they will be deposited around your waist and hips as fat!

So prepare in advance, enjoy the tasty, quick and nutritious meals in this chapter, and lose weight easily.

Chilli Scallops

Shellfish are an excellent source of the essential mineral selenium (apart from their multitude of other nutritional qualities) which our bodies need to make one of the body's own powerful antioxidant enzymes. As we have seen with prawns, the flavours of chillis and shellfish are complementary, but this recipe is equally successful – with a different flavour obviously – omitting the chilli.

For 2

2 tbsp extra-virgin olive oil
75 grams spring onions, chopped into 3–4 cm lengths
1 garlic clove, peeled and chopped finely
1 medium green chilli (or a small red chilli, if you
    prefer really hot!), deseeded and chopped finely
400 gram tin of chopped plum tomatoes
2 tsp tomato purée
2 tbsp dry sherry
1 tbsp chopped fresh oregano
1 tbsp chopped fresh basil

pinch of rock salt
freshly ground black pepper
50 grams butter
8 small scallops, cleaned
200 grams fresh spinach leaves

- Heat the olive oil in a wok and sauté the spring onions, garlic and chilli for 1–2 minutes
- Add the tomatoes, tomato purée, and sherry, season to taste, and simmer gently for 6–8 minutes.

At the same time

- Melt the butter in a small saucepan.
- Separate the orange corals from the scallops, slice the scallops into rounds horizontally, and gently sauté the scallops (and corals) for 3–4 minutes.
- Remove from the pan with a perforated spoon, cover, and set aside.
- Lightly steam the spinach for 2–3 minutes.
- Stir the oregano and basil into the tomato-chilli mixture, add the scallops, and simmer gently for 2–3 minutes.
- Serve immediately on a bed of spinach, garnished with fresh oregano.

CARBOHYDRATE CONTENT PER SERVING: 12 GRAMS

Cauliflower Cheese with Herbs

The humble cauliflower is a rich source of vitamin C, potassium, iron and folate.

For 2

1 medium cauliflower, trimmed to large florets
25 grams of unsalted butter
25 grams of plain flour
250 ml full-cream milk

75 grams of freshly grated cheese of choice (Cheddar,
   such as Red Leicester, or for variety try Orkney,
   Gruyère, Jarlsberg or Edam)
1 tbsp chopped fresh chives
1 tbsp chopped fresh flat-leaf parsley
pinch of rock salt
freshly ground black pepper
freshly chopped chives, to garnish

- Lightly steam the cauliflower florets, and transfer to
  a grill-safe dish.
- Melt the butter in a medium saucepan, remove from
  the heat and stir in the flour.
- Return to a low heat and gradually stir in the milk.
- As the sauce begins to thicken, stir in the grated
  cheese and herbs, and season to taste.
- When the cheese has melted, pour over the
  cauliflower, and place under a medium grill until the
  cheese turns golden, then serve immediately,
  garnished with chopped chives.

CARBOHYDRATE CONTENT PER SERVING: 23 GRAMS

Cod with Olive and Caper Sauce

Olives have been part of a healthy Mediterranean diet
for thousands of years. The ancient Greeks may not
have known that olives are a rich source of
magnesium, vitamin E and the antioxidant polyphenols,
simply that olives have a marvellous taste and
complement many foods.

For 2

2 cod steaks, about 150–175 grams each
25 grams of butter, cubed
pinch of rock salt
freshly ground black pepper

2 tbsp extra-virgin olive oil
1 small red onion, peeled and chopped finely
1 garlic clove, peeled and chopped finely
4 black olives, rinsed and chopped
1 tbsp capers, rinsed and chopped
3 large plum tomatoes, peeled and chopped
1 tsp chopped fresh oregano
sprigs of fresh oregano, to garnish

- Place the cod steaks in the base of an oven-safe baking dish.
- Dot with butter cubes, season to taste, cover with pierced aluminium foil and bake in the centre of a pre-heated oven at 180°C (gas 4) for 12–15 minutes.
- Remove the steaks with a perforated spoon, and place on warm plates.
- While the cod is cooking in the oven, heat the virgin olive oil in a medium frying pan and sauté the onion and garlic for 2–3 minutes.
- Stir in the olives, capers, tomatoes and oregano, and season to taste.
- Simmer gently for 4–5 minutes, then serve the sauce over the baked cod, garnished with fresh oregano.

CARBOHYDRATE CONTENT PER SERVING: 7 GRAMS

Pepper Pork with Ginger

Meat is low in vitamin C, and high in vitamin B. Red and yellow peppers are high in vitamin C. The nutritional combination is obvious, and tastes delicious.

For 2

3 tbsp extra-virgin olive oil
175–200 grams of lean pork fillet, sliced into thin strips
1 medium red onion, peeled and chopped finely

1 garlic clove, peeled and chopped finely
2 slices of fresh ginger root, peeled and chopped
   finely
1 medium red pepper, deseeded and sliced finely
1 medium yellow pepper, deseeded and sliced finely
1 tsp freshly ground black pepper
1 tbsp oyster sauce
1 tbsp sweet sherry
1 tbsp chopped fresh coriander
fresh basil leaves, to garnish

- Heat 2 tbsp of extra-virgin olive oil in a wok and stir-fry the pork strips for 2–3 minutes.
- Remove with a perforated spoon, cover and set aside.
- Heat the remaining tbsp of olive oil in the wok, and sauté the onion and garlic for 1–2 minutes.
- Add the ginger, sweet peppers, freshly ground black pepper, oyster sauce and sherry.
- Stir-fry for 2–3 minutes, then add the coriander and return the pork to the wok.
- Heat through and serve, garnished with fresh basil leaves.

CARBOHYDRATE CONTENT PER SERVING: 19 GRAMS

Beefburgers with Herbs

There is no such thing as a boring hamburger! The potential variations are almost infinite. You can use beef, lamb, pork or turkey mince, and vary the herbs (or omit the herbs) according to taste. The only part you leave out on a low-carbohydrate diet is the bun – and as that has the least taste, it's the least important.

For 2

250 grams of lean mince
   (beef, lamb, pork or turkey)

1 small red onion, diced finely
1 small garlic clove, chopped finely
1 tbsp chopped fresh basil
1 tsp chopped fresh coriander
1 tsp Worcestershire sauce
1 medium free-range egg, beaten
pinch of rock salt
freshly ground black pepper
2 tbsp extra-virgin olive oil
green salad with herbs (page 252)

- Mix together the mince, onion, garlic, basil, coriander, Worcestershire sauce and egg in a large mixing bowl, preferably by hand (definitely the best way for making hamburgers), and season to taste.
- Divide into 4 roughly equal pieces, then roll each into a ball, and pat gently to slightly flatten.
- Chill in the fridge for 1–2 hours.
- Heat the virgin olive oil in a medium frying pan, and cook the hamburgers for about 8 minutes (but vary according to individual taste), turning once.
- Serve immediately with green salad with herbs.

CARBOHYDRATE CONTENT PER SERVING: 2 GRAMS
(WITHOUT SALAD); 3 GRAMS (WITH SALAD)

Stir-fried Turkey with Spicy Mayonnaise

The delicious combination of poultry with creamy curry mayonnaise has been known for decades. This recipe is quick and healthy, so ideal for the cook in a hurry!

For 2

curry mayonnaise with crème fraîche
(page 272)
3 tbsp extra-virgin olive oil

185

300 grams of turkey breast, sliced into thin strips
75 grams of sugarsnap peas
75 grams of French beans
4 spring onions, chopped into 3–4 cm lengths
1 garlic clove, peeled and chopped finely
2 slices of fresh root ginger, peeled and chopped
  finely
1 medium orange pepper, deseeded and sliced thinly
pinch of rock salt
freshly ground black pepper

- Prepare the curry mayonnaise.
- Heat 2 tbsp of extra-virgin olive oil in a wok and stir-fry the strips of turkey breast for 4–5 minutes over moderate heat.
- Remove from the wok, cover, and set aside.
- Heat the remaining virgin olive oil and stir-fry the sugarsnap peas, French beans, spring onions, garlic and ginger for 2–3 minutes.
- Add the pepper and return the turkey to the wok.
- Season to taste, and stir-fry for a further 2–3 minutes.
- Serve immediately, topped with curry mayonnaise.

CARBOHYDRATE CONTENT PER SERVING: 9 GRAMS
(INCLUDING THE MAYONNAISE)

Lamb with Bok Choy

Bok choy is an excellent source of many essential nutrients: beta-carotenes, vitamin B, vitamin C, folate and potassium.

For 2

3 tbsp extra-virgin olive oil
1 tsp sesame oil
200 grams lean lamb, sliced into thin strips

1 red onion, peeled and sliced finely
1 garlic clove, peeled and sliced finely
2 slices of fresh ginger root, peeled and chopped fincly
1 small yellow pepper, deseeded and sliced
1 small red pepper, deseeded and sliced
1 tbsp oyster sauce
1 tbsp light soy sauce
2 tbsp dry sherry
1 tsp caster sugar
pinch of rock salt
freshly ground black pepper
$1/2$ a bok choy (approximately 200 grams), shredded
fresh coriander leaves, to garnish

- Heat 2 tbsp of extra-virgin olive oil in a wok and stir-fry the lamb for 3–4 minutes.
- Remove from the wok with a perforated spoon, cover and set aside.
- Heat the remaining olive oil and sesame oil in the wok, and sauté the onion and garlic for 1–2 minutes.
- Add the ginger, peppers, oyster sauce, soy sauce, sherry and sugar and season to taste.
- Stir-fry for 2–3 minutes, then add the bok choy, return the lamb to the wok, and cook for a further 3 minutes on medium heat.
- Serve immediately, garnished with fresh coriander leaves.

CARBOHYDRATE CONTENT PER SERVING: 12 GRAMS

Prawn Fu-yung

Prawns, herbs, free-range eggs and sherry merge delectably together here. Sherry adds a delicious flavour to the recipe – but no alcohol! In cooking, alcohol boils at a lower temperature than water, so the alcohol evaporates, but the flavour remains.

For 2

3 tbsp extra-virgin olive oil
3 large free-range eggs, beaten
3 spring onions, washed and chopped finely
$\frac{1}{2}$ garlic clove, peeled and chopped finely
150 grams cooked prawns, peeled
2 tsp chopped fresh coriander leaves
1 tbsp dry sherry
freshly ground black pepper
pinch of paprika, to garnish

- Heat 1 tbsp of olive oil in a wok, and scramble the eggs lightly, so that they are still slightly 'runny'.
- Transfer to a bowl, and cover.
- Heat the remaining olive oil, sauté the spring onions and garlic for about a minute, then add the prawns and stir-fry for another minute.
- Add the sherry and coriander, season to taste, stir in the scrambled eggs, and cook for another minute.
- Sprinkle over a pinch of paprika, and serve immediately.

CARBOHYDRATE CONTENT PER SERVING: 2 GRAMS

Fillet Steak with Mushroom Sauce

Button mushrooms have the dietary advantage of a lower carbohydrate content than many other varieties, and the nutritional advantage of providing vitamin B, potassium, phosphorus, sulphur and folate.

For 2

2 tbsp extra-virgin olive oil
2 fillet or eye fillet steaks, approximately
    125–150 grams each; no more than 2.5 cm thick
freshly ground black pepper

75 grams mangetout
75 grams yellow squash

Mushroom sauce

50 grams unsalted butter
1 small red onion, peeled and diced
1 garlic clove, peeled and chopped finely
200 grams button mushrooms, wiped
1 tbsp dry sherry
60 ml chicken stock
1 tbsp chopped fresh chives
75 ml single cream
freshly ground black pepper

- Brush the steak fillets with extra-virgin olive oil on both sides and grill under medium heat (8–10 cm from the grill) for about 6 8 minutes, turning once.

At the same time

- Melt the butter in a medium frying pan and sauté the onion and garlic for 2–3 minutes.
- Add the mushrooms, and sauté for a further 3–4 minutes.
- Stir in the sherry, stock, and chives, season to taste, and simmer gently for 3–4 minutes.
- Add the cream and heat through gently, then pour over the steak.
- Serve with lightly steamed mangetout and yellow squash.

CARBOHYDRATE CONTENT PER SERVING: 9 GRAMS

Coconut Chicken with Pine Nuts

Ready in minutes, this tastes delicious and is high in healthy antioxidants.

For 2

2 skinless chicken breasts, about 150 grams each
1 tbsp freshly squeezed lemon juice
2 tbsp extra-virgin olive oil
1 garlic clove, peeled and chopped finely
3 spring onions, chopped finely
1 yellow pepper, deseeded and sliced finely
30 grams of pine nuts, crushed
1 tbsp chopped fresh basil
1 tbsp chopped fresh flat-leaf parsley
2 plum tomatoes, chopped
50 ml coconut milk
2–3 drops Tabasco sauce (optional)
pinch of rock salt
freshly ground black pepper
chopped fresh chives, to garnish

- Drizzle the lemon juice over the chicken.
- Heat the virgin olive oil in a wok and brown the chicken.
- Stir in the garlic, spring onions, pepper and pine nuts, and stir-fry over medium heat for 2–3 minutes.
- Add the basil, parsley, tomatoes, coconut milk and Tabasco sauce if desired, and season to taste.
- Simmer gently for 10 minutes.
- Serve immediately, garnished with chopped fresh chives.

CARBOHYDRATE CONTENT PER SERVING: 9 GRAMS

Pork and Orange

Vitamin B from pork and vitamin C from orange. Once again, nutrition and flavour complement one another perfectly!

For 2

1 bok choy, halved lengthways
2 tbsp extra-virgin olive oil
200 grams lean pork fillet, sliced thinly
2 shallots, peeled and chopped finely
2 slices of fresh ginger root, peeled and chopped finely
1 medium red pepper, deseeded and sliced finely
2 tsp orange zest
1 tsp honey
freshly ground black pepper
2 tsp chopped fresh chives, to garnish

- Lightly steam the bok choy.
- Heat the extra-virgin olive oil in a wok and stir-fry the pork and shallots for 2–3 minutes, stirring frequently.
- Add the ginger, pepper, orange zest and honey.
- Season to taste, and stir-fry over medium heat for a further 3–4 minutes.
- Place half of the bok choy on each plate, and serve the pork and orange, garnished with chopped chives.

CARBOHYDRATE CONTENT PER SERVING: 11 GRAMS

Crab with Crème Fraîche

Crab has a very 'rich' flavour, and is certainly rich in nutrients, so only a little is necessary. The flavours of crab and herbs need only the simplicity of crème fraîche to bind them, figuratively and gastronomically!

For 2

100 grams of white crab meat, pre-cooked
1 tbsp crème fraîche
1 spring onion, chopped finely
1 tsp chopped fresh basil
1 tsp chopped fresh coriander
2 tsp freshly squeezed lemon juice
pinch of cayenne pepper
150 grams of wild rocket

- Mix together the crab, crème fraîche, spring onion, herbs, lemon juice and cayenne pepper in a medium bowl, and cool in the fridge for 1–2 hours.
- Serve on a base of wild rocket.

CARBOHYDRATE CONTENT PER SERVING: 4 GRAMS
(INCLUDING SALAD)

Steak and Onions

It is impossible to improve upon the taste in this easily prepared, but highly nutritious, meal.

For 2

3 tbsp extra-virgin olive oil
2 portions of frying steak (rump, sirloin or fillet), approximately 150 grams each
1 medium brown onion, peeled and sliced thinly
1 medium red onion, peeled and sliced thinly
1 garlic clove, peeled and chopped finely
75 grams button mushrooms, wiped and sliced
pinch of rock salt
freshly ground black pepper
75 grams French beans

- Heat the virgin olive oil in a medium frying pan and sear the steaks over high heat, then add the onions and garlic, lower the heat and cook to taste:

3–4 minutes for rare, 4–6 minutes for medium, and 6–8 minutes for well-done. Obviously the time of cooking depends on the heat of the pan and the thickness of the steaks.

- After 2–3 minutes, add the mushrooms and season to taste.
- As the steaks are cooking, lightly steam the French beans, and serve immediately.

CARBOHYDRATE CONTENT PER SERVING: 7 GRAMS

Chicken Chop Suey

Once again, poultry with peppers is virtually the perfect nutritional and gastronomic combination, providing most of our essential nutritional requirements. And again, the perfect combination of healthy nutritious food only takes minutes to prepare and cook.

For 2

3 tbsp extra-virgin olive oil
200 grams skinless chicken breast, sliced into thin strips
1 tsp sesame oil
1 garlic clove, peeled and chopped finely
1 slice of fresh ginger root, peeled and chopped finely
75 grams spring onions, chopped into 4–5 cm lengths
1 small yellow pepper, deseeded and sliced
1 small red pepper, deseeded and sliced
75 grams mangetout
2 tbsp light soy sauce
2 tbsp sweet sherry
100 grams beansprouts
freshly ground black pepper

- Heat 2 tbsp extra-virgin olive oil in the wok and stir-fry the chicken strips for 3–4 minutes.
- Remove from the wok with a perforated spoon, set aside and cover.
- Heat the remaining virgin olive oil and sesame oil and sauté the garlic, ginger and spring onions for 1–2 minutes.
- Add the peppers, mangetout, soy sauce, sherry and beansprouts. Season to taste, and stir-fry for 2–3 minutes.
- Return the chicken to the wok and cook over medium heat for a final 2–3 minutes, and serve immediately.

CARBOHYDRATE CONTENT PER SERVING: 8 GRAMS

Pepper Haddock with Mustard Sauce

Peppercorns were once more valuable than gold! Apart from their unique complementary flavour to food, they are also a rich source of chromium. It's certainly impossible to imagine cooking without pepper.

For 2

3 tbsp extra-virgin olive oil
2 haddock fillets, approximately 150–175 grams each
1 tbsp whole black peppercorns, freshly crushed
sprigs of fresh dill, to garnish
crispy green salad (page 248)

Sauce

3 tbsp extra-virgin olive oil
1 tbsp white wine vinegar
1 garlic clove, peeled and chopped finely
2 tsp freshly squeezed lemon juice
1 tsp Dijon mustard

1 tbsp chopped fresh dill
pinch of rock salt
freshly ground black pepper

- Place the crushed black peppercorns on a plate.
- Brush the haddock with extra-virgin olive oil and press the haddock fillets on the pepper to coat thoroughly.
- Grill under medium heat, no closer than 8 cm from the grill, for 5–6 minutes, turning once.

At the same time

- Add the ingredients of the vinaigrette sauce to a screw-top jar and shake well.
- Transfer to a small saucepan and heat through gently.
- Place the haddock on warm plates, pour over the sauce, and garnish with sprigs of fresh dill.
- Serve with crispy green salad.

CARBOHYDRATE CONTENT PER SERVING: 2 GRAMS

Japanese-style Pork

Although an 'ancient' vegetable – whose name originates from the ancient port of Ascalon in Palestine – shallots have all of the healthy properties of their modern relative, the onion. And incidentally, it's not commonly realized that mangetout is a very rich source of vitamin C – almost the same amount as lemons. Mother was right again: eat your greens! Of course, it's much easier (and tastier) if the 'greens' are mangetout, not boiled cabbage.

For 2

3 tbsp extra-virgin olive oil
1 tsp sesame oil

200 grams of lean pork fillet, sliced thinly
2 shallots, peeled and quartered
1 small red pepper, deseeded and sliced thinly
1 small yellow pepper, deseeded and sliced thinly
75 grams mangetout
freshly ground black pepper

Sauce

3 tbsp mirin (Japanese sweet wine)
3 tbsp saké (Japanese rice wine)
4 tbsp shoyu (Japanese soy sauce) (don't use
   Chinese soy sauce – too strong!)
$1/2$ garlic clove, peeled and grated

- Grate the garlic with a ginger- or garlic-grater.
- Mix the ingredients of the sauce in a small bowl,
  then pour half into each of 2 small finger bowls.
- Heat 2 tbsp extra-virgin olive oil and 1 tsp sesame oil
  in a wok and gently stir-fry the pork strips for
  3–4 minutes, stirring frequently.
- Remove from the wok with a perforated spoon, set
  aside and cover.
- Heat the remaining olive oil in the wok and stir-fry
  the vegetables for 3–4 minutes over a moderate heat.
- Return the pork to the wok and heat through for
  about a minute, then serve onto warm plates.
- Place a finger bowl of dipping sauce on each plate.

CARBOHYDRATE CONTENT PER SERVING: 12 GRAMS

Scallops with Honey and Orange Vinaigrette

Iron from scallops and spinach, vitamin C from spinach
and orange, and essential protein and minerals from
scallops: a perfect nutritional and gastronomic
combination!

For 2

30 grams butter
4 large scallops
100 grams of fresh spinach
honey and orange vinaigrette (page 267)

- Prepare the vinaigrette.
- Melt the butter in a small saucepan.
- Separate the corals from the scallops, slice the scallops into rounds horizontally, and gently sauté the scallops (and corals) for 4–5 minutes.
- Remove with a perforated spoon.

Just before the scallops are ready

- Lightly steam the spinach.
- Serve the scallops on a bed of spinach, and drizzle over the honey and orange vinaigrette.

CARBOHYDRATE CONTENT PER SERVING: 14 GRAMS

Herb Chicken Burgers

This recipe proves that real fast food is really healthy – especially burgers. Although chicken forms the basis of the recipe, as all meat and poultry have all the essential amino acids we need, you can use turkey, pork, beef, lamb – even venison, if you prefer! Obviously the taste is different for each, but the nutritional value is the same.

For 2

3 tbsp extra-virgin olive oil
2 shallots, peeled and diced finely
1 garlic clove, peeled and chopped finely
200 grams lean chicken, minced
$1/2$ tbsp chopped fresh basil

$^1/_2$ tbsp chopped fresh coriander
freshly ground black pepper
1 egg white
fennel and tomato salad (page 250)

- Heat 1 tbsp of olive oil in a small saucepan and sauté the shallots and garlic for 1–2 minutes.
- Set aside to cool.
- Mix together the chicken, shallots, garlic, basil and coriander in a medium bowl, and season to taste.
- Add the egg white, stirring thoroughly to bind the mixture.
- Form the mixture into 2 burgers, and cool in the fridge for 30–40 minutes.

At the same time

- Prepare the fennel and tomato salad.
- Heat the remaining 2 tbsp olive oil in a frying pan and cook the burgers for 9–10 minutes, turning once.
- Serve with fennel and tomato salad.

CARBOHYDRATE CONTENT PER SERVING: 13 GRAMS
(1 GRAM WITHOUT SALAD!)

Stir-fried Lamb with Oyster Sauce
Spring onions have all of the healthy attributes of the onion family, and their essential nutrients are retained by gentle stir-frying.

For 2

3 tbsp extra-virgin olive oil
1 tsp sesame oil
200 grams lean lamb fillet, sliced finely
4 spring onions, chopped into 3–4 cm lengths
1 garlic clove, peeled and chopped finely
2 slices of fresh ginger root, peeled and chopped finely

1 small red pepper, deseeded and sliced finely
1 small yellow pepper, deseeded and sliced finely
1 small green pepper, deseeded and sliced finely
1 tbsp oyster sauce
2 tbsp sweet sherry
freshly ground black pepper
finely chopped spring onion, to garnish

- Heat 2 tbsp of extra-virgin olive oil and the sesame oil in a wok and stir-fry the lamb for 2–3 minutes, then remove with a perforated spoon, set aside and cover.
- Heat the remaining olive oil in the wok and add the spring onions, garlic, ginger and peppers.
- Stir-fry for about 2 minutes, then stir in the oyster sauce and sweet sherry.
- Season to taste, return the lamb to the wok, and stir-fry for a final 2 minutes.
- Serve immediately, garnished with finely chopped spring onion.

CARBOHYDRATE CONTENT PER SERVING: 11 GRAMS

Tiger Prawns with Ginger and Garlic

The nutritional value of prawns, ginger and garlic is obvious; less obvious is the nutritional importance of crème fraîche, both for providing essential nutrients like vitamin D and, equally important, to satisfy hunger and slow the digestive process – making us much less likely to needlessly 'snack' on junk food and ruin our diet.

For 2

3 tbsp extra-virgin olive oil
75 grams spring onions, chopped finely
1 garlic clove, peeled and chopped finely

3 slices of fresh ginger root, peeled and chopped
    finely
200 grams cooked tiger prawns, shelled and deveined
1 tbsp sweet sherry
1 tbsp chopped fresh basil
freshly ground black pepper
150 ml crème fraîche
1 tbsp chopped fresh chives, to garnish

- Heat the extra-virgin olive oil in a wok, and lightly sauté the spring onions and garlic for 1–2 minutes.
- Stir in the ginger, prawns, sherry and basil, and season to taste.
- Stir-fry for 2–3 minutes, add the crème fraîche and gently heat through for 1–2 minutes.
- Serve immediately, garnished with chopped fresh chives.

CARBOHYDRATE CONTENT PER SERVING: 5 GRAMS

Peppered Salmon Steaks with Lime

The king of fish is an important source of essential omega-3 fatty acids, and should be included in every healthy diet. But unfortunately even the king of fish is deficient in vitamin C. The rich taste of salmon is complemented by many diverse flavours and nutrients; citrus fruits are an excellent accompaniment, in both taste and nutrition, with their rich source of vitamin C.

For 2

2 salmon steaks, approximately 150–175 grams
    each, approximately 2 cm thick
juice of a freshly squeezed lime
2 tbsp extra-virgin olive oil
2–3 tbsp freshly crushed black peppercorns
caper and olive salad (page 253)
1 tbsp chopped fresh dill and lime zest, to garnish

- Sprinkle a little lime juice over the salmon steaks.
- Brush the steaks with olive oil.
- Place the crushed black peppercorns on a plate and press the salmon steaks on the pepper to cover liberally.
- Cook under a medium grill for 3–4 minutes per side, brushing with olive oil on turning.
- Serve immediately with caper and olive salad.
- Garnish with fresh dill and lime zest.

CARBOHYDRATE CONTENT PER SERVING: 11 GRAMS

Chicken and Ginger

Cashew nuts provide a rich source of zinc, selenium, magnesium, iron and thiamin. As chicken is rich in essential amino acids and other vitamins of the B group, and red pepper is rich in vitamins A and C, this dish is nutritionally perfect!

For 2

3 tbsp extra-virgin olive oil
2 skinless chicken breast fillets, sliced thinly on the diagonal
3 spring onions, chopped into 3–4 cm lengths
1 garlic clove, peeled and chopped finely
3 slices of fresh ginger root, peeled and chopped finely
75 grams mangetout
1 medium red pepper, deseeded and sliced finely
25 grams raw cashew nuts
1 tbsp light soy sauce
1 tbsp dry sherry
freshly ground black pepper
2 tsp chopped fresh chives

- Heat 2 tbsp of extra-virgin olive oil in a wok and stir-fry the chicken for 3–4 minutes.
- Remove with a perforated spoon, and set aside.
- Heat the remaining tbsp of olive oil in the wok, and sauté the spring onions and garlic for 1–2 minutes.
- Add the ginger, mangetout, pepper, cashew nuts, soy sauce and sherry, and season to taste.
- Stir-fry for 2–3 minutes, then return the chicken to the wok and cook for a further 2–3 minutes.
- Serve immediately, garnished with freshly chopped chives.

CARBOHYDRATE CONTENT PER SERVING: 12 GRAMS

Calamari with Basil and Coriander

This recipe is another example of how quick and easy it is to produce delicious and very healthy meals with simple – but healthy – ingredients. The secret lies in the content: food that is good for you almost always tastes good! With fresh calamari, extra-virgin olive oil, basil and coriander, it's just not possible to find any healthier foods. This is a perfect entrée.

For 2

200 grams fresh calamari tubes, chopped into 1 cm rings
2 tbsp extra-virgin olive oil
2 tbsp freshly squeezed lemon juice
1 garlic clove, peeled and chopped finely
3 spring onions, chopped finely
1 tbsp chopped fresh basil leaves
1 tsp chopped fresh coriander leaves
freshly ground black pepper
fresh basil leaves, to garnish

- Place the calamari in a saucepan of boiling water, reduce the heat and simmer for about 4–5 minutes.
- Set aside to cool.
- Mix together the extra-virgin olive oil and lemon juice, stir in the calamari, and marinate for 6–8 hours in the fridge.
- Prior to serving, stir in the garlic, spring onions and herbs. Season to taste, and garnish with fresh basil leaves.

CARBOHYDRATE CONTENT PER SERVING: 1 GRAM

Liver with Basil

Liver is one of the most nutritious of all foods. And it provides more vitamin C than lemons!

For 2

3 tbsp extra-virgin olive oil
300 grams lamb's liver, sliced finely
2 medium red onions, peeled and sliced thinly
1 garlic clove, peeled and chopped finely
1 tbsp plain flour
100 ml lamb stock
pinch of rock salt
freshly ground black pepper
75 ml single cream
1 tbsp chopped fresh basil
75 grams carrot, julienne
75 grams of broccoli florets
fresh basil leaves, to garnish

- Heat the extra-virgin olive oil in a large frying pan and braise the liver for about a minute on each side.
- Add the onions and garlic, and gently sauté for about 3–4 minutes.

- Remove from the heat and stir in the flour, then gradually add the stock, stirring constantly.
- Season to taste, bring to the boil, then lower the heat and gently simmer for 8–10 minutes.
- Remove from the heat and stir in the cream and basil, then heat through gently.
- Serve immediately with lightly steamed broccoli and julienne carrots, garnished with fresh basil leaves.

CARBOHYDRATE CONTENT PER SERVING: 14 GRAMS

Piperade

There are many variations on this popular dish, essentially because the basic concept – like all good food – is amenable to minor variation in ingredients without compromising taste and quality in any way. Eggs are incredibly nutritious, providing essential amino acids, vitamins A, D, B_2, B_{12}, folate, phosphorus and iodine.

For 2

2 large plum tomatoes, peeled, deseeded and diced
25 grams butter
1 medium red onion, peeled and diced
1 garlic clove, peeled and chopped finely
1 medium green pepper, deseeded and diced
1 medium yellow pepper, deseeded and diced
1 tsp chopped fresh basil
4 large free-range eggs, beaten
freshly ground black pepper
50 grams freshly grated Edam cheese
fresh basil leaves, to garnish

- Place the tomatoes in a small bowl of boiling water for about 15–20 seconds, then rinse under cold water.

- The tomatoes can then be easily peeled, de-seeded and diced.
- Melt the butter in a medium frying pan and gently sauté the onions and garlic for 2–3 minutes.
- Stir in the tomatoes and peppers, and cook over low heat for 8–10 minutes.
- Add the eggs, sprinkle over the basil and season to taste.
- When the eggs are almost cooked, sprinkle over the cheese, and place under a hot grill until the cheese melts. (The cheese is optional, but adds immensely to the flavour.)
- Serve immediately, garnished with fresh basil leaves.

CARBOHYDRATE CONTENT PER SERVING: 7 GRAMS

Salmon with Bok Choy

Bok choy has a delightful texture and unique flavour. It complements salmon perfectly, especially with a light soy dressing. But be careful never to overcook the bok choy, or its intrinsic nutrition will be lost in cooking. Overcooking is the certain way to destroy natural nutrition in healthy food.

For 2

2 salmon steaks, about 150–175 grams each
25 grams of butter, cubed
2 slices of fresh ginger root, peeled and sliced julienne
2 bok choy, quartered vertically
freshly ground black pepper
sprigs of fresh dill, to garnish

Dressing

1 tbsp light soy sauce

1 tbsp sweet sherry
$\frac{1}{2}$ tsp sesame oil
$\frac{1}{2}$ tsp grated fresh root ginger

- Mix together the soy sauce, sweet sherry, sesame oil and grated ginger, and set aside.
- Place the salmon steaks in the base of an ovenproof dish, top with ginger strips, and dot with cubes of butter.
- Cover with pierced aluminium foil, and bake in the centre of a pre-heated oven at 180°C (gas 4) for about 20 minutes, depending on the oven.

Just before the salmon is ready

- Lightly steam the bok choy (3–4 minutes is sufficient).
- Transfer the salmon to the plates with a perforated spoon.
- Place the bok choy adjacent to the salmon.
- Drizzle the dressing over the bok choy.
- Finally, garnish with sprigs of fresh dill.

CARBOHYDRATE CONTENT PER SERVING: 1 GRAM

Crab with Spicy Mayonnaise

Shellfish are a rich source of iodine, which is essential for the functioning of our thyroid glands. Without iodine in the diet, your metabolism slows down, and so do you!

For 2

3 tbsp mayonnaise – fresh (page 268) or commercial
200 grams fresh white crabmeat, pre-cooked
1 tsp curry powder
pinch of cayenne pepper
chopped fresh chives, to garnish
red lettuce salad (page 254)

- Mix together the mayonnaise, crabmeat, curry powder and cayenne pepper in a small bowl.
- Cover, and chill in the fridge for 3–4 hours (optional).
- Garnish with chopped fresh chives, and serve with red lettuce salad – without dressing.

CARBOHYDRATE CONTENT PER SERVING: 11 GRAMS (INCLUDING THE SALAD); < 1 GRAM (WITHOUT THE SALAD)

Parma Ham and Parmesan Frittata

Parma ham is a rich source of essential amino acids and vitamins, especially thiamin (vitamin B_1), which combines perfectly, both gastronomically and nutritionally, with the taste (and vitamin D) of Parmesan and eggs.

For 2

4 large free-range eggs, beaten
1 large plum tomato, peeled and chopped
2 tsp chopped fresh oregano
100 grams Parma ham, chopped finely
50 grams Parmesan cheese, grated
pinch of rock salt
freshly ground black pepper
2 tbsp extra-virgin olive oil
2 spring onions, chopped finely
1 garlic clove, peeled and chopped finely
red lettuce salad (page 254)

- Mix together the eggs, tomato, oregano, Parma ham and Parmesan cheese, reserving some cheese to garnish, and season to taste.
- Heat the extra-virgin olive oil in a medium frying pan, and gently sauté the spring onions and garlic for 2–3 minutes.

- Add the egg mixture and cook over low heat for about 10 minutes, until almost set.
- Garnish with freshly grated Parmesan, and place under a low grill for 1–2 minutes.
- Serve with red lettuce salad.

CARBOHYDRATE CONTENT PER SERVING: 3 GRAMS
(WITHOUT SALAD); 14 GRAMS (WITH SALAD)

Poached Whiting with Ginger

Whiting has all of the essential amino acids naturally present in fish, with a deliciously sweet flavour that combines beautifully with fresh ginger. Lemon juice adds an essential zest to the recipe, and the missing vitamin C!

For 2

4 medium whiting fillets, about 75 grams each
julienne strips of ginger and spring onion, to garnish
8 baby leeks

Sauce

100 ml full-cream milk
2 tbsp sweet sherry
1 tbsp light soy sauce
1 garlic clove, peeled and grated
2 slices of fresh ginger root, peeled and grated
pinch of rock salt
freshly ground black pepper
2 tsp freshly squeezed lemon juice

- Mix together the ingredients of the sauce.
- Place the fillets in a single layer in the base of a large frying pan, and pour over the sauce.
- Bring to the boil, then reduce the heat to a gentle simmer for about 10–12 minutes.

Just before the whiting is ready

- Lightly steam the baby leeks for 3–4 minutes.
- Serve the whiting (pouring any remaining sauce over the fish) with the baby leeks.
- Garnish with julienne ginger and spring onion.

CARBOHYDRATE CONTENT PER SERVING: 5 GRAMS

Chilli Turkey

One of the most popular misconceptions is that you have to use beef mince (which is excellent, but not essential) for chilli. Turkey mince has a unique flavour which blends with the hot chilli powder.

For 2

2 tbsp extra-virgin olive oil
350 grams turkey mince
1 large brown onion, peeled and sliced
1 garlic clove, peeled and chopped finely
1 tsp chilli powder
1 tsp ground cumin
400 gram tin of chopped plum tomatoes
100 ml chicken stock
1 bay leaf
2 tsp chopped fresh oregano
pinch of rock salt
freshly ground black pepper
75 grams mangetout
75 grams sugarsnap peas

- Heat the virgin olive oil in a medium frying pan and brown the turkey mince (although it doesn't really 'brown' like beef mince).
- Stir in the onion and garlic, and sauté for 1–2 minutes.

- Stir in the chilli powder, cumin, plum tomatoes (plus juice), chicken stock, bay leaf and fresh oregano.
- Season to taste and simmer gently for 10–15 minutes.

At the same time

- Lightly steam the mangetout and sugarsnap peas.
- Serve the chilli turkey with the vegetables.

CARBOHYDRATE CONTENT PER SERVING: 14 GRAMS

Oysters au Naturel

When discussing recipes for health, one must never forget that simplicity is essential. Oysters are the perfect example where any intervention by the over-zealous cook will inevitably spoil the taste and nutrition. Apart from being a marvellous source of all essential amino acids, they are also high in iodine, phosphorus and zinc – not to mention their aphrodisiac properties, of course! They are undoubtedly best enjoyed au naturel, chilled with perhaps (but not essentially) a few drops of freshly squeezed lemon juice.

For 2

12 (or 24!) fresh oysters, chilled
freshly squeezed lemon juice (optional)

- Shell the oysters (the tricky part), sprinkle over a few drops of lemon juice, if desired, and enjoy.

CARBOHYDRATE CONTENT PER SERVING: NEGLIGIBLE

Tuna with Bok Choy

This meal can be prepared and cooked in a matter of minutes. It tastes delicious, and provides a very nutritious lunch or light supper. Few people realise that peppers are one of the richest sources of vitamin C – more than either oranges or lemons!

For 2

2 tbsp extra-virgin olive oil
2 shallots, peeled and quartered lengthways
1 garlic clove, peeled and chopped finely
1 slice of fresh ginger root, peeled and chopped finely
1 bok choy, trimmed and sliced
1 yellow pepper, deseeded and sliced thinly
1 tbsp light soy sauce
2 tbsp dry sherry
200 gram tin of tuna (in brine or springwater), drained
freshly ground black pepper
finely chopped spring onion, to garnish

- Heat the extra-virgin olive oil in the wok and sauté the shallots and garlic for 1–2 minutes.
- Stir in the ginger, bok choy, pepper, soy sauce and sherry, and stir-fry for 2–3 minutes.
- Add the tuna, season to taste, and stir-fry for a final 2 minutes.
- Serve immediately, garnished with finely chopped spring onion.

CARBOHYDRATE CONTENT PER SERVING: 3 GRAMS

Soufflé Omelette

Eggs are an excellent source of vitamin B$_{12}$, which is essential for the function of blood cells.

The pepper can be replaced by lightly steamed asparagus (chopped finely) or chopped spring onion.

For 2

4 large free-range eggs, separated
75 grams Gruyère cheese (or Emmental, Edam, or
    Jarlsberg . . . or whatever cheese you prefer)
2 tbsp full-cream milk
1 small red pepper, deseeded and diced finely
pinch of rock salt
freshly ground black pepper
50 grams unsalted butter
1 tbsp chopped fresh basil, to garnish

- Beat the egg yolks in a medium bowl.
- Stir in the cheese, milk and pepper, and season to taste.
- Beat the egg whites until stiff, and gradually 'fold' into the egg yolk mixture.
- Heat the butter in a medium omelette pan, add the omelette mixture, and cook over a low heat for about 5–7 minutes.
- Sprinkle over grated Gruyère cheese, and grill under a pre-heated grill for about a minute.
- Serve immediately, garnished with chopped fresh basil.

CARBOHYDRATE CONTENT PER SERVING: 3 GRAMS

Char-grilled Tuna Steaks

Simply delicious and totally nutritious! This has to be the ultimate 10-minute meal – and so healthy. Char-grilled tuna can be served with a salad, as suggested, or with either lightly steamed or stir-fried vegetables. Tuna is usually served rare, but can be cooked for longer if you prefer it more thoroughly cooked.

For 2

3 tbsp extra-virgin olive oil
2 tuna steaks, approximately 150–175 grams each
freshly ground black pepper
rocket and olive salad (page 247)

- Brush the tuna steaks with olive oil, sprinkle with freshly ground black pepper, and char-grill for 5–6 minutes, turning once.
- Serve with rocket and olive salad.

CARBOHYDRATE CONTENT PER SERVING: 1 GRAM
(INCLUDING SALAD!)

Shellfish Omelette

This meal is best described as somewhere between an omelette and a frittata, as the omelette is cooked through, then sliced; it can be enjoyed either hot or cold, and is therefore ideal as a light meal which can be prepared in advance.

For 2

4 large fresh free-range eggs
2 tbsp full-cream milk
100 grams cooked prawns, shelled and deveined
100 grams cooked white crabmeat, flaked
1 tbsp chopped fresh coriander
1 tsp chopped fresh chives
2–3 drops of Tabasco sauce
pinch of rock salt
freshly ground black pepper
2 tbsp extra-virgin olive oil
fresh coriander leaves, to garnish

213

- Beat together the eggs and milk in a medium bowl, and add the prawns, crab, coriander, chives and Tabasco sauce. Season to taste.
- Heat the olive oil in a large frying pan, and add the mixture, ensuring that the mixture evenly covers the base of the frying pan.
- Cook over medium heat.
- When the omelette has almost set, it can be folded (as usual) and served, garnished with fresh coriander leaves, or it can be allowed to set until just firm, then removed and sliced. The latter can be served hot or cold.

CARBOHYDRATE CONTENT PER SERVING: 2 GRAMS

Swordfish with Basil and Coriander

Simple and incredibly nutritious; yet another example of how easy it is to provide real fast food which also happens to be healthy!

For 2

2 swordfish steaks, approximately 150–175 grams each
2 tsp chopped fresh coriander
1 tbsp chopped fresh basil
pinch of rock salt
freshly ground black pepper
balsamic vinaigrette (page 266)
crispy green salad (page 248)

- Cook the swordfish steaks under a hot grill for 2–3 minutes per side, approximately 8–10 cm from the grill.
- Transfer to warm plates and sprinkle over the fresh coriander and basil.

- Season to taste, drizzle over balsamic vinaigrette (not too much!) and serve immediately with crispy green salad.

CARBOHYDRATE CONTENT PER SERVING: NEGLIGIBLE

Garlic Prawns

Garlic and chilli is a heavenly – and healthy – combination. With the aromatic delicate flavour of fresh dill, this makes a delicious entrée, or light supper.

For 2

75 grams butter
3 garlic cloves, peeled and chopped finely
1 small green chilli, chopped finely (optional)
200 grams uncooked tiger prawns, shelled and deveined
1 tbsp chopped fresh dill
freshly ground black pepper
sprigs of fresh dill, to garnish

- Melt the butter in a medium saucepan and sauté the garlic and chilli for 1–2 minutes.
- Stir in the prawns, cook for 3–4 minutes.
- Stir in the chopped dill and pepper.
- Garnish with sprigs of fresh dill and serve immediately.

CARBOHYDRATE CONTENT PER SERVING: NEGLIGIBLE

Chapter 7

Vegetarian Meals, Vegetables and Salads

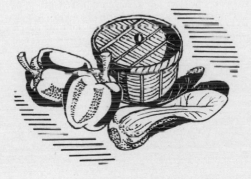

All vegetables are healthy, but unfortunately some vegetables (particularly root vegetables) have a relatively high carbohydrate content. Obviously, these are 'good' carbohydrates, as distinct from the 'bad' refined carbohydrates, such as sugars, cakes, biscuits, sweets, white rice, pasta and bread. But unfortunately our body cannot distinguish between 'good' and 'bad' carbohydrates in depositing fat, so we have to omit the high-carbohydrate vegetables in a weight-loss diet. All of the essential vitamins and minerals which they contain are provided by other elements of the diet.

It is certainly possible, but quite complicated, to ensure a healthy high-protein, low-carbohydrate intake on a vegetarian diet. Unfortunately, there is neither the time or space available in this book to achieve this aim, however the following recipes will nutritionally complement a diet including meat, poultry, fish and shellfish.

The nutrition in vegetables is superb, with particularly high levels of vitamins and minerals, but no vegetable or fruit contains *all* of the essential amino acids, which are the 'building blocks' of body proteins, unlike meat, poultry and fish which do contain all essential amino acids. As it is our intention to keep the diet as easy-to-follow as possible, and ensure healthy weight loss, meat and fish are an essential component of this diet.

Asparagus with Parmesan Herb Sauce

Asparagus is a rich source of copper, magnesium and calcium, as well as vitamins A, B_2, C and E.

For 2

400 grams asparagus, washed and trimmed
50 grams melted butter
1 medium red onion, peeled and diced
1 medium red pepper, deseeded and sliced finely
2 tbsp breadcrumbs, grated finely
30 grams freshly grated Parmesan cheese
4 large plum tomatoes, peeled and chopped thickly
1 tbsp chopped fresh oregano
1 tbsp chopped fresh basil
pinch of rock salt
freshly ground black pepper
fresh basil leaves, to garnish

- Place the asparagus lengthways in the base of a baking dish and pour over the melted butter.
- Mix together the onion, pepper, breadcrumbs, cheese, tomatoes and freshly chopped herbs, and season to taste.
- Pour the mixture over the asparagus, cover and bake in a pre-heated oven at 180°C (gas 4) for 25-30 minutes.
- Serve immediately, garnished with fresh basil leaves.

CARBOHYDRATE CONTENT PER SERVING: 19 GRAMS

Aubergine and Pepper

Although aubergines and peppers are both members of the potato family, they could not have originated further apart geographically: peppers were brought to Europe by Columbus from the west, and aubergines made their way across Asia (slowly) from India. But their combined flavours are delightful.

For 2

2 tbsp extra-virgin olive oil
3 baby onions, peeled and quartered lengthways
1 garlic clove, peeled and chopped finely
1 medium aubergine, sliced
1 medium red pepper, deseeded and sliced
   horizontally
2 large plum tomatoes, quartered lengthways
1 tbsp tomato purée
50 ml Chardonnay
1 tbsp chopped fresh basil leaves
pinch of rock salt
freshly ground black pepper
fresh oregano leaves, to garnish

- Place the sliced aubergine in a colander, sprinkle with salt, and allow to stand for 20–30 minutes, then rinse thoroughly and pat dry.
- Heat the extra-virgin olive oil in a medium frying pan and sauté the onions and garlic for 2–3 minutes, then add the aubergine, pepper and tomatoes, and gently sauté for 3–4 minutes.
- Stir in the tomato purée, Chardonnay and fresh basil leaves, season to taste, and simmer for 5–7 minutes.
- Serve immediately, garnished with fresh oregano leaves.

CARBOHYDRATE CONTENT PER SERVING: 10 GRAMS

Baby Onions with Mushrooms and Garlic

Thyme has been recognized for its antibiotic qualities for centuries, and is an excellent companion to the other antioxidants (in onions, ginger, and garlic) for good health.

For 2

3 tbsp extra-virgin olive oil
1 tsp sesame oil
8 baby onions, peeled
2 garlic cloves, peeled and chopped finely
2 slices of fresh ginger root, peeled and chopped
75 grams button mushrooms, wiped
1 tsp chopped fresh rosemary
1 tsp chopped fresh thyme
freshly ground black pepper
sprigs of fresh rosemary, to garnish

- Heat the extra-virgin olive oil and sesame oil in a large frying pan and sauté the onions and garlic for 2–3 minutes.
- Add the ginger, mushrooms, rosemary and thyme, season to taste, and cook for a further 3–4 minutes.
- Serve immediately, garnished with sprigs of fresh rosemary.

CARBOHYDRATE CONTENT PER SERVING: 6 GRAMS

Bok Choy with Oyster Sauce

This is a simple and quick vegetable side-dish that complements many main courses.

For 2

2 tbsp extra-virgin olive oil
$\frac{1}{2}$ tsp sesame oil

1 slice of fresh ginger root, peeled and chopped
   finely
1 bok choy, shredded
1 tbsp oyster sauce
freshly ground black pepper

- Heat the extra-virgin olive oil and sesame oil in the wok and sauté the ginger and bok choy for about a minute.
- Stir in the oyster sauce, season to taste, and stir-fry for a further 2 minutes.

CARBOHYDRATE CONTENT PER SERVING: 3 GRAMS

Chilli Aubergine

Aubergines have the capacity to absorb flavours, particularly herbs and spices, better than virtually any other vegetable.

For 2

1 large aubergine, sliced
rock salt
3 tbsp extra-virgin olive oil
2 large plum tomatoes, chopped
1 garlic clove peeled and chopped finely
1 medium green pepper, deseeded and chopped
2 spring onions, chopped finely
1 medium green chilli, deseeded and chopped finely
1 tbsp chopped fresh coriander
freshly ground black pepper
fresh coriander leaves, to garnish

- Place the aubergine slices in a colander, sprinkle with salt, and allow to stand for 20–30 minutes, then rinse thoroughly and pat dry.
- Heat 2 tbsp of extra-virgin olive oil in a large frying pan, and brown the aubergine slices.

- Remove the slices from the pan, dry on kitchen paper, and chop into large chunks.
- Heat the remaining olive oil, add the tomatoes, garlic, green pepper, spring onions and chilli, and sauté for 3–4 minutes.
- Return the aubergine pieces to the pan, stir in the coriander, season to taste and cook over medium heat for 2–3 minutes.
- Serve immediately, garnished with fresh coriander leaves.

CARBOHYDRATE CONTENT PER SERVING: 5 GRAMS

Leeks with Coriander

Leeks are actually members of the onion family, and therefore contain many of the essential nutrients present in onions.

For 2

2 tbsp extra-virgin olive oil
1 tbsp unsalted butter
8 baby leeks, trimmed
2 large plum tomatoes, peeled, deseeded and chopped
1 medium garlic clove, peeled and chopped finely
1 tbsp sweet sherry
2 tsp freshly squeezed lemon juice
1 tbsp chopped fresh coriander
freshly ground black pepper
fresh coriander leaves, to garnish

- Heat the extra-virgin olive oil and butter in a medium saucepan and sauté the leeks for 5–7 minutes.
- Add the tomatoes, garlic, sherry, lemon juice and coriander, season with freshly ground black pepper,

and simmer gently for about 5 minutes, stirring occasionally.
- Serve immediately, garnished with fresh coriander.

CARBOHYDRATE CONTENT PER SERVING: 6 GRAMS

Broccoli with Oyster Sauce

All kinds of broccoli are nutritious, but the green and purple varieties have the highest content of calcium and folate.

For 2

- Follow the recipe Bok Choy with Oyster Sauce (page 224), substituting bok choy with 250 grams of broccoli florets.

CARBOHYDRATE CONTENT PER SERVING: 3 GRAMS

Brussels Sprouts with Chilli and Ginger Sauce

Brussels sprouts are a very rich source of vitamin C – almost twice the content of oranges – and are an excellent source of folate.

For 2

200 grams Brussels sprouts, trimmed and
    'crossed' at base
chilli and ginger sauce (page 274)
freshly ground black pepper
2 sprigs of fresh thyme, to garnish

- Lightly steam the Brussels sprouts.
- Season to taste, pour over the chilli and ginger sauce, and garnish with sprigs of fresh thyme.

CARBOHYDRATE CONTENT PER SERVING: 19 GRAMS

Caponata

This is a delicious variation on the well-known Italian dish, providing a rich source of antioxidants from virtually every ingredient.

For 4

1 large aubergine, cubed
rock salt
3 tbsp extra-virgin olive oil
1 large red onion, peeled and sliced
2 garlic cloves, peeled and chopped finely
1 medium red pepper, deseeded and sliced
1 medium yellow pepper, deseeded and sliced
1 celery stick, chopped into 2–3 cm pieces
2 large green courgettes, chopped into large pieces
    on the diagonal
400 grams plum tomatoes, peeled and chopped (or
    400 gram tin of chopped plum tomatoes)
1 tbsp chopped fresh basil leaves
1 tbsp chopped fresh chives
1 tbsp capers, drained and rinsed
2 tsp granulated sugar
75 ml red wine vinegar
50 grams green olives
pinch of rock salt
freshly ground black pepper
fresh basil leaves, to garnish

- Place the aubergine cubes in a colander, sprinkle with salt and leave for 20–30 minutes, then rinse with cold water and pat dry.
- Heat the extra-virgin olive oil in a medium frying pan and sauté the onion and garlic for 1–2 minutes.
- Add the peppers and celery, and cook for a further 2 minutes, then add the aubergine and courgettes.

- Cook on low heat for 3–4 minutes, then stir in the tomatoes, and gently simmer for about 10 minutes.
- Add the basil, chives, capers, sugar, red wine vinegar and olives.
- Season to taste, and gently simmer for a final 4–5 minutes before serving.
- Garnish with fresh basil leaves.

CARBOHYDRATE CONTENT PER SERVING: 11 GRAMS

Char-grilled Vegetables with Sesame Seeds

Char-grilling is a very healthy method of cooking, retaining almost all of the nutrition in the vegetables.

For 2

1 small green pepper, deseeded and
    quartered lengthways
1 small red pepper, deseeded and quartered
    lengthways
2 small red onions, peeled and quartered lengthways
2 large plum tomatoes, quartered lengthways
4 yellow squash, halved lengthways
2 tbsp extra-virgin olive oil
freshly ground black pepper
1 tsp sesame seeds
fresh basil leaves, to garnish

- Dry stir-fry the sesame seeds for about a minute, then set aside.
- Arrange the vegetables in a single layer, skin uppermost, on a metal grill-tray, brush with extra-virgin olive oil, and grill under medium heat, approximately 8 cm from the grill, for 7–8 minutes.
- Remove from the grill, and peel the skin from the peppers, onions and tomatoes.

- Season to taste, and sprinkle lightly toasted sesame seeds over the vegetables.
- Serve immediately, garnished with fresh basil leaves.

CARBOHYDRATE CONTENT PER SERVING: 12 GRAMS

Fennel and Herbs with Swiss Cheese

Fennel imparts a delightful aniseed flavour to food, and provides an excellent source of potassium and calcium, as well as vitamins A and E.

For 2

2 fennel bulbs
1 tbsp chopped fresh basil
1 tbsp chopped fresh chives
freshly ground black pepper
75 grams butter, melted
25 grams grated Gruyère cheese
25 grams grated Emmental cheese
fresh basil leaves and chopped chives, to garnish

- Top-and-tail the fennel bulbs, cut into segments vertically, and lightly steam until cooked.
- Place the fennel in a grill-safe dish, sprinkle with fresh chopped basil and chives, season to taste, then pour over the melted butter.
- Mix together the Gruyère and Emmental cheese, sprinkle the mixture evenly over the fennel, then grill until the cheese has melted.
- Serve immediately, garnished with fresh basil leaves and chopped chives.

CARBOHYDRATE CONTENT PER SERVING: 6 GRAMS

Green Vegetables and Oyster Sauce

Spring onions are merely the young shoots of the onion, and therefore have all of the health-giving properties of the parent plant.

For 2

2 tbsp extra-virgin olive oil
1 tsp sesame oil
4 spring onions, washed and chopped into 3–4 cm lengths
1 garlic clove, peeled and chopped finely
2 slices of fresh ginger root, peeled and chopped finely
1 small green pepper, deseeded and sliced
75 grams broccoli florets
small bunch of asparagus (approximately 100 grams), trimmed and chopped into 3–4 cm lengths
1 tbsp oyster sauce
1 tbsp sweet sherry
pinch of rock salt
freshly ground black pepper
chopped fresh chives, to garnish

- Heat the extra-virgin olive oil and sesame oil in the wok, and sauté the spring onions and garlic for 1–2 minutes.
- Stir in the ginger, pepper, broccoli, asparagus, oyster sauce and sherry.
- Season to taste, and stir-fry for 3–4 minutes.
- Serve immediately, garnished with fresh chopped chives.

CARBOHYDRATE CONTENT PER SERVING: 6 GRAMS

Baby Leeks in Basil Sour Cream

Leeks provide the antioxidants carotene and vitamin E, and both iron and folate which are so essential for healthy blood cells.

For 2

8 baby leeks, trimmed
pinch of rock salt
freshly ground black pepper
100 grams sour cream
1 tbsp chopped fresh basil
pinch of paprika, to garnish

- Lightly steam the seasoned baby leeks.
- Stir the fresh basil into the sour cream.
- Top the leeks with the basil sour cream, and garnish with paprika.

CARBOHYDRATE CONTENT PER SERVING: 4 GRAMS

Aubergine with Courgettes

Courgettes are an excellent source of minerals (potassium and iron) and the antioxidant vitamins A and C.

For 2

3 tbsp extra-virgin olive oil
1 medium aubergine, cubed
1 tsp sesame oil
3 spring onions, chopped into 3-4 cm lengths
1 garlic clove, peeled and chopped finely
2 slices of fresh ginger root, peeled and chopped finely
4 large courgettes, chopped on the diagonal
4 large plum tomatoes, chopped
2 tbsp light soy sauce
1 tbsp sweet sherry

pinch of rock salt
freshly ground black pepper

- Place the aubergine cubes in a colander, sprinkle with salt, and allow to stand for 20-30 minutes, then rinse thoroughly and pat dry.
- Heat 2 tbsp of extra-virgin olive oil in a large frying pan, and brown the aubergine cubes.
- Remove from the pan and pat dry.
- Heat the remaining virgin olive oil and the sesame oil in the wok and gently sauté the spring onions and garlic for 2-3 minutes.
- Stir in the ginger, courgettes, tomatoes, soy sauce and sherry, and season to taste.
- Return the aubergine to the pan and stir-fry for 5-7 minutes over moderate heat, and serve immediately.

CARBOHYDRATE CONTENT PER SERVING: 13 GRAMS

Mushrooms with Garlic

Mushrooms are a very rich source of the mineral zinc, which is essential for the production of one of the body's natural antioxidant enzymes, 'superoxide dismutase'.

For 2

3 tbsp extra-virgin olive oil
1 medium red onion, peeled and sliced
2 garlic cloves, peeled and chopped finely
200 grams of button mushrooms, wiped
1 tbsp chopped fresh chives
1 tbsp chopped fresh coriander
1 tbsp freshly squeezed lemon juice
freshly ground black pepper
fresh coriander leaves, to garnish

- Heat the extra-virgin olive oil in a wok and gently sauté the onion and garlic for 1–2 minutes.
- Add the mushrooms, and sauté for a further 3–4 minutes, stirring constantly.
- Stir in the chives and coriander, add the lemon juice, and season to taste.
- Garnish with fresh coriander leaves.

CARBOHYDRATE CONTENT PER SERVING: 5 GRAMS

Peppers with Herbs

This recipe provides vitamins A, C and E from the peppers and even more healthy antioxidants from the herbs.

For 4

2 medium yellow peppers, deseeded and quartered
2 medium red peppers, deseeded and quartered
2 medium orange peppers, deseeded and quartered

Marinade

4 tbsp extra-virgin olive oil
1 tbsp white wine vinegar
1 tbsp chopped fresh flat-leaf parsley
1 tbsp chopped fresh coriander
1 tbsp chopped fresh basil
freshly ground black pepper

- Mix together the ingredients of the marinade in a medium bowl.
- Char-grill the peppers according to the method on page 265, then remove the skin and slice finely.
- Stir the pepper slices into the marinade, cover and chill in the fridge for 3–4 hours before serving.

CARBOHYDRATE CONTENT PER SERVING: 7 GRAMS

Mushrooms with Rosemary and Thyme Cream Sauce

Button mushrooms contain about a quarter of the carbohydrate content of oyster mushrooms, and are particularly useful in a low-carbohydrate diet, especially as the nutritional content is identical.

For 2

3 tbsp extra-virgin olive oil
75 grams shallots, peeled and chopped
1 garlic clove, peeled and chopped finely
200 grams of button mushrooms, trimmed, wiped
   and halved
2 tsp chopped fresh rosemary
2 tsp chopped fresh thyme
pinch of rock salt
pinch of cayenne pepper
100 ml crème fraîche
sprigs of fresh thyme, to garnish

- Heat the extra-virgin olive oil in a wok and gently sauté the shallots and garlic for 2-3 minutes.
- Stir in the mushrooms, rosemary and thyme, and season to taste.
- Stir-fry on medium heat for 3-4 minutes, then remove from the heat and stir in the crème fraîche.
- Heat through gently and serve immediately, garnished with fresh thyme.

CARBOHYDRATE CONTENT PER SERVING: 4 GRAMS

Spicy Vegetables

Mangetout is a variety of pea, not bean, and provides a particularly rich source of vitamin C, in addition to potassium, calcium and phosphorus.

For 2

3 tbsp extra-virgin olive oil
1 medium red onion, peeled and sliced
1 garlic clove, peeled and chopped finely
100 grams of broccoli florets
50 grams of mangetout
50 grams of French beans
1 tsp ground cumin
1 tsp ground fennel seeds
1 tbsp chopped fresh coriander
$1/2$ tsp garam masala
1 slice of fresh ginger root, peeled and chopped
   finely
100 ml of chicken stock
100 grams of spinach, chopped
1 tbsp freshly squeezed lemon juice
1 tbsp dry sherry
pinch of rock salt
freshly ground black pepper

- Heat the extra-virgin olive oil in a wok and sauté the
  onion and garlic for 1–2 minutes.
- Add the broccoli, mangetout and French beans, and
  stir-fry for 2–3 minutes.
- Stir in the cumin, fennel, coriander, garam masala
  and ginger, and cook for about a minute, then add
  the chicken stock and simmer for 4–5 minutes.
- Stir in the spinach, lemon juice and sherry, season
  to taste, and simmer for a final 2 minutes before
  serving.

CARBOHYDRATE CONTENT PER SERVING: 6 GRAMS

Asparagus with Lemon Butter Sauce

Asparagus has been considered an aphrodisiac since
Roman times!

For 2

200 grams asparagus, washed and trimmed
75 grams butter
juice of $1/2$ a freshly squeezed lemon
freshly ground black pepper
fresh basil leaves, to garnish

- Lightly steam the asparagus.
- Melt the butter in a small saucepan, stir in the
  lemon juice, and season to taste.
- Arrange the asparagus on warm plates, pour over the
  lemon butter sauce, and garnish with fresh basil.

CARBOHYDRATE CONTENT PER SERVING: 4 GRAMS

Stir-fried Vegetables

Dry-toasting the sesame seeds releases the distinctive
nut-like flavour and aroma locked within the husk.

For 2

1 tbsp sesame seeds
2 tbsp extra-virgin olive oil
1 tsp sesame oil
2 small red onions, quartered lengthways
1 garlic clove, peeled and chopped finely
2 slices of fresh ginger root, peeled and chopped
    finely
1 small red pepper, deseeded and sliced finely
1 small yellow pepper, deseeded and sliced finely
75 grams broccoli florets
75 grams mangetout

75 grams button mushrooms, wiped and halved
2 tbsp light soy sauce
2 tbsp sweet sherry
freshly ground black pepper

- Lightly toast the sesame seeds in a dry pan for about a minute, and set aside.
- Heat the extra-virgin olive oil and sesame oil in the wok and sauté the onion and garlic for 1–2 minutes.
- Add the ginger, peppers, broccoli, mangetout and mushrooms.
- Stir in the soy sauce and sherry, season to taste, and stir-fry for 3–4 minutes.
- Serve immediately, garnished with the toasted sesame seeds.

CARBOHYDRATE CONTENT PER SERVING: 14 GRAMS

Sweet Chestnuts with Crème Fraîche and Basil

Sweet chestnuts have a higher carbohydrate content than many other nuts, but can still be included in a low-carbohydrate diet, in moderation. Their nutritional content is as high as all nuts, and the flavour quite unique.

For 2

150 grams of fresh sweet chestnuts
15 grams of butter
pinch of rock salt
freshly ground black pepper
75 grams of crème fraîche
1 tbsp chopped fresh basil
fresh basil leaves, to garnish

- Make a slit in the shell of each chestnut very carefully; ensure you support the chestnut on the chopping board, and <u>never</u> cut towards yourself, as it is too easy for the blade to slip and cause a nasty cut.

- Place the pierced chestnuts in a pan of cold water, bring to the boil, then lower the heat and simmer for about 5 minutes.
- Remove with a perforated spoon, and cool under running cold water.
- Peel the shells carefully with a knife.
- Place the peeled chestnuts in a medium saucepan with the butter, and season to taste.
- Add sufficient water to lightly cover the chestnuts, bring to the boil, then lower the heat and simmer for about 25–30 minutes until the chestnuts are tender, then drain the chestnuts.
- Mix the crème fraîche with the basil, spoon onto the chestnuts, and garnish with fresh basil.

CARBOHYDRATE CONTENT PER SERVING: 28 GRAMS

Char-grilled Aubergines with Peppers

Onions have immense nutritional qualities, apart from their value as an excellent source of minerals, such as potassium, calcium, iron and phosphorus.

For 2

2 finger aubergines, quartered lengthways
1 small red pepper, deseeded and quartered
  lengthways
1 small yellow pepper, deseeded and quartered
  lengthways
1 small red onion, quartered lengthways
1 garlic clove, peeled and grated
2 tbsp extra-virgin olive oil
pinch of rock salt

freshly ground black pepper
fresh coriander leaves, to garnish

Dressing

4 tbsp extra-virgin olive oil
1 tbsp balsamic vinegar
1 tsp Dijon mustard
1 garlic clove, peeled and grated
pinch of rock salt
freshly ground black pepper
1 tbsp chopped fresh coriander

- Grate the garlic with a ginger- or garlic-grater.
- Add the ingredients of the dressing to a screw-top jar and shake well to mix thoroughly.
- Arrange the vegetables in a single layer, skin uppermost, on a metal grill-tray, brush with extra-virgin olive oil, and sprinkle over the grated garlic.
- Grill under medium heat, approximately 8 cm from the grill, for 7–8 minutes.
- Remove from the grill, and peel the skins from the peppers and onion.
- Season to taste, drizzle over the dressing, and serve immediately, garnished with fresh coriander leaves.

CARBOHYDRATE CONTENT PER SERVING: 8 GRAMS

Vegetable Goulash

Unusually, the content of the powerful antioxidant lycopene is higher in cooked tomatoes than in their fresh form.

For 2

1 tbsp extra-virgin olive oil
1 garlic clove, peeled and chopped finely
1 tbsp flour
1 tbsp ground paprika

200 ml chicken stock
400 gram tin of chopped plum tomatoes
4 baby onions, peeled
150 grams broccoli florets
150 grams carrots, peeled and sliced into matchsticks
100 grams cauliflower florets
1 small red pepper, deseeded and sliced
1 small green pepper, deseeded and sliced
3–4 drops of Tabasco sauce
pinch of rock salt
freshly ground black pepper
1 tbsp chopped fresh oregano
1 tbsp chopped fresh basil
100 ml sour cream
1 tbsp chopped fresh chives, to garnish
75 grams French beans
75 grams mangetout

- Heat the extra-virgin olive oil in a medium frying pan, and sauté the garlic for a minute.
- Remove from the heat, and stir in the flour and paprika.
- Return to the heat, and stir in the tomatoes and stock.
- Add the onions, broccoli, carrots, cauliflower, peppers and Tabasco sauce, season to taste, and simmer for 5 minutes.
- Transfer to an oven-safe casserole dish, and cook in the centre of a pre-heated oven at 190°C (gas 5) for 20–25 minutes.
- Stir in the oregano and basil and return to the oven for 10 minutes.
- Remove from the oven, stir in the sour cream lightly to achieve a 'marbled' effect, and garnish with chopped chives.
- Serve with lightly steamed French beans and mangetout.

CARBOHYDRATE CONTENT PER SERVING: 22 GRAMS

Spinach with Chilli and Pine Nuts

Nuts are an excellent source of the essential antioxidant vitamin E.

For 2

200 grams of spinach
2 tbsp pine nuts, lightly toasted
2 tbsp extra-virgin olive oil
2 spring onions, chopped into 3–4 cm lengths
1 garlic clove, peeled and chopped finely
1 small red chilli, deseeded and chopped finely (optional)
pinch of rock salt
freshly ground black pepper
lemon and coriander vinaigrette (page 267)

- Lightly steam the spinach for 3–4 minutes, and set aside.

At the same time

- Lightly toast the pine nuts in a dry pan, and set aside.
- Heat the extra-virgin olive oil in a small frying pan and gently sauté the spring onions, garlic and chilli for 3–4 minutes.
- Mix together the spinach, pine nuts, spring onions, garlic and chilli, and season to taste.
- Drizzle over lemon and coriander vinaigrette.

CARBOHYDRATE CONTENT PER SERVING: 3 GRAMS

Baked Peppers with Mozzarella

Ideal as a light snack or supper dish, an excellent combination of vitamin A and vitamin C from peppers, and vitamin D from Mozzarella.

For 4

2 tbsp extra-virgin olive oil
2 medium onions, peeled and chopped finely
2 garlic cloves, peeled and chopped finely
2 tsp tomato purée
4 large vine-ripened tomatoes, peeled and diced
1 tbsp chopped fresh oregano
freshly ground black pepper
4 large yellow peppers, deseeded and top removed
2 slices of prosciutto ham, diced
4 thick slices of Mozzarella cheese
fresh basil leaves, to garnish

- Heat the extra-virgin olive oil in a saucepan and lightly sauté the onion and garlic for 1–2 minutes.
- Stir in the tomato purée.
- Pour the mixture into a bowl, and add the diced tomatoes and oregano.
- Season to taste, and mix thoroughly.
- Spoon the mixture into the peppers, and place the peppers on a baking tray, adding a little water to the tray.
- Cook in the centre of a pre-heated oven at 160°C (gas 2) for 25–30 minutes.
- Remove from the oven, sprinkle over the prosciutto ham, top with slices of Mozzarella cheese, and place under a medium grill for 1–2 minutes, until the cheese has melted.
- Serve immediately, garnished with fresh basil leaves.

CARBOHYDRATE CONTENT PER SERVING: 10 GRAMS

Herb Tomatoes

This is virtually pure antioxidant, from garlic, herbs and tomatoes. No free radicals after this meal!

For 2

1 garlic clove, peeled and chopped finely
1 tbsp of chopped fresh basil
1 tbsp of chopped fresh flat-leaf parsley
2 beefsteak tomatoes, halved
1 tbsp of fresh breadcrumbs
1 tbsp extra-virgin olive oil
pinch of rock salt
freshly ground black pepper
chopped fresh chives, to garnish

- Mix together the garlic, basil and parsley.
- Add 3–4 tbsp water to a shallow casserole dish then place the tomatoes (cut side uppermost) in the dish.
- Place half the garlic and herb mixture on each tomato, top with breadcrumbs, and drizzle a little extra-virgin olive oil on the tomatoes.
- Bake in the centre of a pre-heated oven at 180°C (gas 4) for 10–12 minutes.
- Serve immediately, garnished with chopped chives.

CARBOHYDRATE CONTENT PER SERVING: 11 GRAMS

Aubergine in Coriander Cream Sauce

Aubergines are one of the richest sources of vitamin E, with more than 50 times the concentration in potatoes.

For 2

1 medium aubergine, sliced
rock salt
3 tbsp extra-virgin olive oil
15 grams butter

15 grams plain flour
150 ml full-cream milk
1 tbsp chopped fresh coriander
1 tbsp chopped fresh flat-leaf parsley
freshly ground black pepper
2 tbsp single cream

- Place the aubergine slices in a colander, sprinkle with rock salt and leave for 20–30 minutes. Rinse with cold water and pat dry.
- Heat the virgin olive oil in a medium frying pan and fry the aubergine slices until well-cooked.
- Melt the butter in a small saucepan, remove from the heat and stir in the flour.
- Return to a low heat and gradually blend in the milk, stirring constantly.
- When the sauce begins to thicken, stir in the coriander and parsley, season to taste, and stir in the cream.
- Heat through gently for about 30 seconds, stirring constantly, and serve immediately over the crisp aubergine slices.

CARBOHYDRATE CONTENT PER SERVING: 14 GRAMS

Salads

Avocado with Crème Fraîche

Avocado is another food with an aphrodisiac reputation. Perhaps we should change the title of the book!

For 2

- 1 large ripe Hass avocado, peeled, stoned and cubed
- 1 small red pepper, deseeded and chopped into small cubes

1 small yellow pepper, deseeded and chopped into
   small cubes
1 tbsp chopped fresh chives
1 tbsp chopped fresh basil
150 ml crème fraîche
freshly ground black pepper
2 sprigs of fresh thyme, for garnish

- Mix together the avocado, peppers, chives and basil in a medium bowl.
- Stir in the crème fraîche, season to taste, and garnish with sprigs of fresh thyme.

CARBOHYDRATE CONTENT PER SERVING: 17 GRAMS

Chicken and Cashew Salad

Spinach is rich in vitamins and minerals, but overcooking prevents the absorption of calcium and iron from the spinach, so the maximum nutritional value (and best flavour) is ensured by eating it raw or lightly steamed.

For 2

2 chicken breast fillets, approximately
   100–150 grams each
200 grams spinach leaves, washed
1 Lebanese cucumber, sliced lengthways
3 spring onions, chopped into 4–5 cm lengths
1 small Hass avocado, halved, stoned, peeled and
   sliced thinly
1 tbsp chopped fresh basil
50 grams raw cashew nuts
25 grams pine nuts
freshly ground black pepper
lemon and coriander vinaigrette (page 267)

- Place the chicken fillets in a shallow oven-safe dish and dot with butter.
- Cover with perforated aluminium foil and cook in the centre of a pre-heated oven at 180°C (gas 4) for 40–45 minutes.
- Remove with a perforated spoon and set aside to cool. When cool, slice on the diagonal into 2–3 cm slices.
- Arrange the spinach on the plates. Toss the cucumber, spring onions, avocado and basil with the nuts, and spoon onto the spinach.
- Place the chicken on the salad and drizzle over the dressing.

CARBOHYDRATE CONTENT PER SERVING: 10 GRAMS

Rocket and Olive Salad

Rocket is one of the foods to be 're-discovered' in recent times, but in actual fact there is evidence of its cultivation 10,000 years ago. Unfortunately – or fortunately – its use in recipes has been rather dominated by its aphrodisiac reputation.

For 2

100 grams rocket leaves, washed
2 tsp capers, rinsed
50 grams black olives
3 anchovy fillets, chopped
1 tbsp chopped fresh coriander
1 tbsp freshly squeezed lemon juice
freshly ground black pepper
60 ml balsamic vinaigrette (page 266)

- Mix together the rocket, capers, olives, anchovies, coriander and lemon juice, and season to taste.
- Drizzle over the balsamic vinaigrette.

CARBOHYDRATE CONTENT PER SERVING: 1 GRAM

Coriander Vegetables and Crème Fraîche

Onions are an important source of the mineral 'molybdenum', which is essential for the synthesis of DNA.

For 2

2 tbsp extra-virgin olive oil
100 grams yellow squash, quartered lengthways
1 medium fennel, thinly sliced
6 spring onions, chopped into 3–4 cm lengths
75 grams carrots, julienne
1 garlic clove, peeled and sliced finely
150 ml crème fraîche
1 tbsp chopped fresh coriander
freshly ground black pepper
fresh basil leaves, to garnish

- Heat the extra-virgin olive oil in a wok, and stir-fry the squash, fennel, spring onions, carrots and garlic for 3–4 minutes.
- Mix in the coriander and cook for a further minute.
- Season to taste, and spoon onto plates.
- Top with crème fraîche, and garnish with fresh basil leaves.

CARBOHYDRATE CONTENT PER SERVING: 9 GRAMS

Crispy Green Salad

Lettuce is well-recognized for its high fibre content, but rather less well-known as a source of carotene and vitamin C, and a particularly high source of potassium.

For 2

50 grams wild rocket
100 grams mixed crispy lettuce leaves (coral, green oak, frisee, mizuna, cos)

4 spring onions, chopped into 4–5 cm lengths on the
   diagonal
25 grams mangetout
1 tbsp chopped fresh basil
1 tbsp chopped fresh coriander
fresh basil and coriander leaves, to garnish

- Mix together the ingredients of the salad, and drizzle
  over a dressing of choice.

CARBOHYDRATE CONTENT PER SERVING: NEGLIGIBLE

Roasted Pepper and Bocconcini Salad

If possible, try to use the true Bocconcini, made from
buffalo milk. The difference in taste is well worth the
effort!

For 2

1 medium yellow pepper, deseeded and quartered
1 medium red pepper, deseeded and quartered
2 tbsp extra virgin olive oil
100 grams of Bocconcini cheese, sliced thinly
2 medium vine-ripened tomatoes, sliced
pinch of rock salt
freshly ground black pepper
balsamic vinaigrette (page 266)
fresh basil leaves, to garnish

- Place the peppers in an oven-safe dish, drizzle over
  the extra-virgin olive oil, cover with pierced
  aluminium foil and bake in the centre of a pre-
  heated oven at 180°C (gas 4) for 20–25 minutes.
- Remove from the oven and set aside. When cool,
  slice into thin strips.
- Mix together the peppers and place in the centre of
  the plates.

- Arrange the tomato and Bocconcini slices alternately around the peppers, season to taste, drizzle over the balsamic vinaigrette, and garnish with fresh basil leaves.

CARBOHYDRATE CONTENT PER SERVING: 8 GRAMS

Fennel and Tomato Salad

The aniseed flavour of fennel blends subtly with that of semi-dried tomatoes.

For 2

2 fennel bulbs, trimmed, outer leaves removed, and quartered lengthways
50 grams mangetout
4 spring onions, chopped finely
4 semi-dried tomatoes with herbs (page 254) or sun-dried tomatoes, quartered
1 tbsp chopped fresh coriander
freshly ground black pepper
50 grams rocket
fresh shavings of Parmesan cheese and fresh basil leaves, to garnish

- Lightly steam the quartered fennel bulbs and mangetout, and set aside to cool.
- Mix together the fennel, mangetout, spring onions, tomatoes and coriander.
- Season to taste, and serve on a bed of rocket.
- Garnish with fresh shavings of Parmesan cheese and basil leaves.

CARBOHYDRATE CONTENT PER SERVING: 12 GRAMS

Feta and Olive Salad

This is often described as a Greek salad, but is actually present in many Mediterranean countries.

For 2

2 large plum tomatoes, quartered lengthways
1 Lebanese cucumber, chopped on the diagonal
3 spring onions, chopped into 3–4 cm lengths on the
   diagonal
100 grams of black olives, halved and stoned
100 grams of Feta cheese, cubed
freshly ground black pepper
French vinaigrette (page 266) *or* lemon and coriander
   vinaigrette (page 267)

- Mix together the ingredients of the salad, and dress
  with either a simple vinaigrette, or lemon and
  coriander vinaigrette for extra zest.

CARBOHYDRATE CONTENT PER SERVING: 5 GRAMS

Lebanese Salad

Lebanese cucumber is particularly useful in a low-carbohydrate diet as it has a lower carbohydrate content than the English variety, but the same nutritional value.

For 2

100 grams cooked prawns
100 grams broccoli florets, lightly steamed
1 medium Lebanese cucumber, sliced on the
   diagonal
3 large plum tomatoes, chopped into large cubes
1 tbsp chopped fresh basil
1 tbsp chopped fresh chervil
8–10 black olives, halved and stoned

4 anchovy fillets, sliced thinly
freshly ground black pepper
fresh basil leaves, to garnish
French vinaigrette (page 266)

- Mix the ingredients of the salad in a medium bowl, and season to taste.
- Pour over French vinaigrette, and garnish with fresh basil leaves.

CARBOHYDRATE CONTENT PER SERVING: 13 GRAMS

Green Salad with Herbs

Borage is an excellent source of omega-6 essential fatty acid.

For 2

150 grams of mixed green salad leaves (rocket, watercress, dandelion, baby spinach and fresh borage leaves)
2 tsp chopped fresh basil
2 tsp chopped fresh coriander
2 tsp chopped fresh chervil
pinch of rock salt
freshly ground black pepper
mint and chives vinaigrette (page 266)

- Mix together the green salad leaves, basil, coriander and chervil, and season to taste.
- Drizzle over the mint and chives vinaigrette.

CARBOHYDRATE CONTENT PER SERVING: 2 GRAMS

Caper and Olive Salad

Lycopene from tomatoes, polyphenols in olives, and vitamin E from nuts: a recipe for good health.

For 2

75 grams baby spinach leaves
2 spring onions, chopped into 2–3 cm pieces
2 large plum tomatoes, deseeded and chopped
1 tsp capers, rinsed
4–5 green olives, stoned and halved
4–5 black olives, stoned and halved
1 garlic clove, peeled and grated
25 grams of pine nuts, lightly toasted
2 tsp chopped fresh basil
pinch of rock salt
freshly ground black pepper
passata vinaigrette (page 268)

- Mix together the baby spinach leaves, spring onions, tomatoes, capers, olives, garlic, pine nuts and basil.
- Season to taste and drizzle over the passata vinaigrette.

CARBOHYDRATE CONTENT PER SERVING: 8 GRAMS

Asparagus and Parma Ham Salad

Vitamin B_1 from Parma ham, vitamin D from Parmesan cheese, and vitamin A from asparagus are only some of the essential nutrients provided by this delicious recipe.

For 2

150 grams of asparagus, trimmed
75 grams of rocket
3 slices of Parma ham, sliced finely
1 tbsp chopped fresh chives

30 grams of Parmesan cheese, as shavings
pinch of rock salt
freshly ground black pepper
pine nuts, to garnish
lemon and coriander vinaigrette (page 267)

- Lightly steam the asparagus until tender but still firm.
- Mix together the asparagus, rocket, Parma ham,
  chives and Parmesan, and season to taste.
- Drizzle over lemon and coriander vinaigrette, and
  garnish with pine nuts.

CARBOHYDRATE CONTENT PER SERVING: 2 GRAMS

Red Lettuce Salad

The colour tells you that this recipe is high in
vitamin A!

For 2

100 grams of mixed red lettuce leaves (radicchio, red
   oak lettuce, lollo rosso, mignonette)
1 small red pepper, deseeded and sliced thinly
1 red onion, peeled and sliced thinly
4 semi-dried tomatoes with herbs (below)
1/2 small red chilli, deseeded and chopped finely

- Mix together the ingredients of the salad and drizzle
  over the dressing of choice.

CARBOHYDRATE CONTENT PER SERVING: 11 GRAMS

Semi-dried Tomatoes with Herbs

Tomatoes and thyme are foods with an extremely high
concentration of antioxidants.

For 4

8 large plum tomatoes, quartered lengthways

1 tbsp chopped fresh basil
1 tbsp chopped fresh thyme
freshly ground black pepper
2 tbsp extra-virgin olive oil

- Place the tomatoes skin down on a wire rack in a baking tray, sprinkle with the herbs and pepper, and cook in the centre of a pre-heated oven at 150°C (gas 2) for about 2½–3 hours.
- Remove from the oven and set aside to cool.
- Mix with extra-virgin olive oil, and cool in the fridge for 3–4 hours before use.

CARBOHYDRATE CONTENT PER SERVING: 6 GRAMS

Vegetable Salad

Oriental vinaigrette adds zest to this colourful and nutritious salad.

For 2

75 grams mangetout
50 grams French beans
1 small yellow pepper, deseeded and sliced thinly
1 small red pepper, deseeded and sliced thinly
3 spring onions, chopped into 4–5 cm lengths on the diagonal
3 baby yellow squash, quartered vertically
freshly ground black pepper
oriental vinaigrette (page 268)
lime zest and fresh basil leaves, to garnish

- Lightly steam the vegetables then pour over the dressing.
- Garnish with lime zest and fresh basil leaves.

CARBOHYDRATE CONTENT PER SERVING: 8 GRAMS

Vine-ripened Cherry Tomatoes with Bocconcini and Parmesan

An unusual combination of soft and hard cheeses which blend perfectly together.

For 2

2 tbsp extra-virgin olive oil
2 tomato vines, each of 6 cherry tomatoes
75 grams of wild rocket
75 grams of Boccincini cheese, sliced thinly
50 grams of freshly grated Parmesan cheese
1 small Hass avocado, halved, peeled, stoned and
   chopped
1 tbsp chopped fresh basil leaves
1 tsp chopped fresh coriander leaves
freshly ground black pepper
balsamic vinaigrette (page 266)
fresh basil leaves, to garnish

- Brush the cherry tomatoes (on the vine) with the olive oil, and grill, 8 cm from the heat, for 2 minutes.
- Mix together the rocket, Bocconcini, Parmesan, avocado, basil and coriander, and season to taste.
- Place the warm cherry tomatoes (still on the vine) on the salad, and drizzle over the balsamic vinaigrette.
- Garnish with fresh basil leaves.

CARBOHYDRATE CONTENT PER SERVING: 4 GRAMS

Char-grilled Onions with Herbs

Char-grilling preserves most of the nutrition in vegetables, and is therefore one of the healthiest methods of cooking.

For 2

2 medium brown onions, peeled and quartered
1 tbsp extra-virgin olive oil
2 tsp chopped fresh basil
2 tsp chopped fresh coriander
pinch of rock salt
freshly ground black pepper
balsamic vinaigrette (page 266)
fresh basil leaves, to garnish

* Place the onion quarters in an oven-safe dish,
  sprinkle over the extra-virgin olive oil and herbs, and
  season to taste.
* Cover with pierced aluminium foil and bake in the
  centre of a pre-heated oven at 180°C (gas 4) for
  30–35 minutes.
* Remove from the oven and place under a hot grill
  for 3–4 minutes per side.
* Drizzle over a little balsamic vinaigrette, and serve
  immediately, garnished with fresh basil leaves.

CARBOHYDRATE CONTENT PER SERVING: 5 GRAMS

Chives and Pepper Salsa

The sweet flavour of the peppers with the zest of the
other member of the pepper family, the chilli, provides
a rich source of vitamins A and C.

For 2

2 medium red peppers, deseeded and quartered
1 medium yellow pepper, deseeded and quartered
1 tbsp extra-virgin olive oil
1 garlic clove, peeled and chopped finely
1/2 large green chilli, deseeded and chopped finely
1 tbsp chopped fresh chives

Dressing

> 2 tbsp extra-virgin olive oil
> 1 tsp white wine vinegar
> pinch of rock salt
> freshly ground black pepper

- Add the ingredients of the dressing to a screw-top jar and shake well to mix thoroughly.
- Arrange the peppers in a single layer, skin uppermost, on a metal grill-tray.
- Brush with extra-virgin olive oil and grill under medium heat, approximately 8 cm from the grill, for 7–8 minutes.
- Remove from the grill, and peel the skins from the peppers.
- Allow to cool, then dice finely.
- Mix together the peppers, garlic, chilli and chives.
- Drizzle over the dressing, and season to taste.
- Garnish with fresh coriander leaves before serving.

CARBOHYDRATE CONTENT PER SERVING: 7 GRAMS

Chicken and Bocconcini Salad

Essential amino acids and vitamins from chicken, and protein, calcium and vitamin D from Bocconcini. Not to mention the aphrodisiac properties of rocket.

For 2

> 2 skinless chicken breasts, approximately
>   150 grams each
> 25 grams of butter, cubed
> 100 grams wild rocket
> 100 grams Bocconcini, sliced finely
> 1 small yellow pepper, deseeded and sliced finely
> 8–10 black olives
> red pesto sauce (page 277)

pinch of rock salt
freshly ground black pepper

- Place the chicken breasts in a medium oven-safe casserole dish, dot with butter, cover with pierced aluminium foil and cook in the centre of a pre-heated oven at 180°C (gas 4) for 30–35 minutes. Remove from the oven and set aside to cool before slicing finely.
- Arrange a bed of wild rocket on the plates, place the rounds of Bocconcini and slices of cool chicken on the rocket, sprinkle over the sliced pepper and olives, and drizzle over the red pesto sauce. Season to taste, and serve immediately.

CARBOHYDRATE CONTENT PER SERVING: 8 GRAMS

Chapter 8

Dressings and Sauces

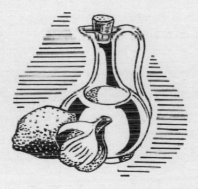

The problem with most diets is that they consist of tasteless polystyrene food, which is virtually inedible, so the diet fails. This is most obvious in the areas of sauces and dressings; low-fat sauces and dressings are usually no-taste sauces and dressings. Even worse, low-fat alternatives are usually high in carbohydrates, so not only do they taste bland, their integral carbohydrates increase your insulin levels and actually *prevent* breakdown of body fat – the opposite effect to that intended. In this diet, you can have delicious sauces and dressings, which are also high in nutritional value, because the reduction in carbohydrate in your diet means that the calories will not be converted to fat. On the contrary, you will continue to lose weight at a safe, steady rate whilst enjoying delicious meals, complemented by delicious sauces and dressings, from gravy and mint sauce on roast meats, to delicious mayonnaises and vinaigrettes for dressings. Most are very quick and simple to prepare, and because they are low in carbohydrate (and high in healthy ingredients) they help to ensure healthy weight loss by complementing a delicious and nutritious diet.

The recipes are not cast in stone. Providing you keep carbohydrates low in your diet, you can adjust recipes to your individual taste. For example, you may prefer a slightly different combination of wine vinegar to olive oil in your vinaigrette, or a different oil. Adjust to your preference; the aim is to provide you with guidelines to delicious eating whilst easily dieting.

Dressings

French Vinaigrette

For 2

4 tbsp extra-virgin olive oil
1 tbsp white wine vinegar
$^1/_2$ tsp mustard powder
$^1/_2$ garlic clove, peeled and chopped finely
pinch of rock salt
freshly ground black pepper

- Add the ingredients of the dressing to a screw-top jar, and shake to mix well.

CARBOHYDRATE CONTENT PER SERVING: NEGLIGIBLE

Balsamic Vinaigrette

For 2

4 tbsp extra-virgin olive oil
1 tbsp balsamic vinegar
$^1/_2$ garlic clove, peeled and chopped finely
pinch of rock salt
freshly ground black pepper

- Place all of the ingredients into a screw-top jar and mix thoroughly.

CARBOHYDRATE CONTENT PER SERVING: NEGLIGIBLE

Mint and Chives Vinaigrette

For 2

5 tbsp extra-virgin olive oil
1 tbsp white wine vinegar
1 tsp dry mustard
$^1/_2$ garlic clove, peeled and chopped finely

2 tsp chopped fresh chives
2 tsp chopped fresh mint
pinch of rock salt
freshly ground black pepper

- Add the ingredients of the vinaigrette to a screw-top jar and mix thoroughly.

CARBOHYDRATE CONTENT PER SERVING: 1 GRAM

Honey and Orange Vinaigrette

For 4

5 tbsp extra-virgin olive oil
1 tbsp white wine vinegar
1 tbsp honey
2 tbsp freshly squeezed orange juice
1 tsp orange zest

- Mix together the ingredients in a screw-top jar and shake well.

CARBOHYDRATE CONTENT PER SERVING: 7 GRAMS

Lemon and Coriander Vinaigrette

For 2

5 tbsp extra-virgin olive oil
1 tbsp white wine vinegar
1 small garlic clove, peeled and chopped finely
1 tbsp freshly squeezed lemon juice
1 tbsp chopped fresh coriander
freshly ground black pepper

- Mix together the ingredients in a screw-top jar and shake thoroughly.

CARBOHYDRATE CONTENT PER SERVING: NEGLIGIBLE

Oriental Vinaigrette

For 2

5 tbsp extra-virgin olive oil
1 tbsp white wine vinegar
1 tbsp light soy sauce
1 tbsp sweet sherry
1 tsp sesame oil
1 slice of fresh ginger root, peeled and chopped
   finely
freshly ground black pepper

- Mix the ingredients in a screw-top jar and shake well.

CARBOHYDRATE CONTENT PER SERVING: 1 GRAM

Passata Vinaigrette

For 2

3 tbsp extra-virgin olive oil
3 tbsp passata (or tomato juice)
1 tbsp red wine vinegar
$^1/_2$ garlic clove, peeled and grated
pinch of rock salt
freshly ground black pepper

- Add the ingredients of the vinaigrette to a screw-top jar and mix well.

CARBOHYDRATE CONTENT PER SERVING: 3 GRAMS

Mayonnaise

For 6

2 egg yolks from large, free-range eggs
1 garlic clove, peeled and chopped finely
1 tsp Dijon mustard
1 tsp white wine vinegar

200 ml extra-virgin olive oil
pinch of rock salt
freshly ground black pepper

- Place the egg yolks, garlic, mustard and white wine vinegar in a food processor and blend for a few seconds, then – with the motor running – add the olive oil slowly and evenly.
- Season to taste, adding a little extra white wine vinegar if necessary.

CARBOHYDRATE CONTENT PER SERVING: NEGLIGIBLE

Aioli (Garlic Mayonnaise)

- Use the same method as above, adding a further 2 garlic cloves to the recipe.

CARBOHYDRATE CONTENT PER SERVING: NEGLIGIBLE

Herb Mayonnaise

For 6

200 ml mayonnaise (page 268)
1 tbsp chopped fresh chives
1 tbsp chopped fresh tarragon
1 tsp chopped fresh coriander

- Prepare the mayonnaise in a blender according to the recipe on page 268.
- Stir in the chives, tarragon and coriander, and check the seasoning.

CARBOHYDRATE CONTENT PER SERVING: NEGLIGIBLE

Hot Mayonnaise

For 4

150 ml mayonnaise (as page 268, or commercial)
1/2 tsp Worcestershire sauce
pinch of cayenne pepper

- Stir the Worcestershire sauce and cayenne pepper into the mayonnaise. If commercial mayonnaise is used, add a tsp of mustard (of choice).

CARBOHYDRATE CONTENT PER SERVING: NEGLIBLE

Chilli Mayonnaise

For 3

1 large red chilli, deseeded and chopped finely
  (replace with a small red chilli if you like it hot!)
1 garlic clove, peeled and chopped finely
1 tsp tomato purée
2–3 drops Tabasco sauce
100 ml mayonnaise (as page 268, or commercial)
pinch of rock salt
freshly ground black pepper
fresh coriander leaves, to garnish

- Add the ingredients to a food processor and blend until smooth.
- Chill for 2–3 hours before serving, garnished with fresh coriander leaves.

CARBOHYDRATE CONTENT PER SERVING: 1 GRAM

Creamy Curry Mayonnaise

For 6

1 tbsp extra-virgin olive oil
$\frac{1}{2}$ small onion, peeled and diced finely
1 small garlic clove, peeled and chopped finely
1 tbsp medium curry powder
75 ml red wine
1 tbsp sweet sherry
1 tsp freshly squeezed lemon juice
1 bay leaf
pinch of rock salt
freshly ground black pepper
200 ml mayonnaise (page 268)
30 ml single cream

- Heat the extra-virgin olive oil in a medium frying pan and gently sauté the onion and garlic for 2–3 minutes.
- Stir in the curry powder and cook for another 2–3 minutes.
- Add the wine, sherry, lemon juice and bay leaf, and season to taste.
- Bring to the boil, lower the heat and gently simmer for about 8–10 minutes, then remove from the heat and set aside to cool.
- When cool, remove the bay leaf and slowly add the sauce to the mayonnaise, stirring constantly.
- When fully combined, add the cream slowly, once again stirring constantly.
- Cool in the fridge for 2–3 hours before serving.

CARBOHYDRATE CONTENT PER SERVING: 2 GRAMS

Curry Mayonnaise with Crème Fraîche

If you need a simple and delicious curry mayonnaise quickly, this solves the problem.

For 2

2 tbsp home-made mayonnaise (page 268), or
    commercial mayonnaise
2¹⁄₂ tbsp crème fraîche
2 tsp Madras curry powder
1 tsp tomato ketchup

- Mix together the ingredients and chill in the fridge for 1–2 hours before serving.

CARBOHYDRATE CONTENT PER SERVING: 2 GRAMS

Sauces

Basic White Sauce

For 4

20 grams plain flour
30 grams butter
200 ml full-cream milk
freshly ground black pepper (optional)

- Melt the butter in a small saucepan, remove from the heat and blend in the flour.
- Return to a low heat and slowly add the milk, stirring constantly.
- Season to taste.

CARBOHYDRATE CONTENT PER SERVING: 7 GRAMS

Béchamel Sauce

For 4

200 ml full-cream milk
1 slice of onion
blade of mace
5 black peppercorns
1 bay leaf
20 grams plain flour
30 grams butter
pinch of rock salt
freshly ground black pepper

- Add the onion, mace, peppercorns, bay leaf and milk to a small saucepan, and gently heat through for 8–10 minutes.
- Remove from the heat and strain the milk.
- Using the infused milk, make the white sauce according to the method on page 272.

CARBOHYDRATE CONTENT PER SERVING: 8 GRAMS

Basil and Chive Sauce

For 4

200 ml béchamel sauce (above)
1 tbsp chopped fresh basil
1 tbsp chopped fresh chives

- Prepare the béchamel sauce, as above.
- Stir in the chopped fresh basil and chives, and serve immediately.

CARBOHYDRATE CONTENT PER SERVING: 8 GRAMS

Leek and Lemon Butter Sauce

For 4

1 medium leek
100 grams butter
2 tbsp freshly squeezed lemon juice
1 tbsp chopped fresh basil
freshly ground black pepper

- Lightly steam the leek, and chop into 1–2 cm segments.
- Melt the butter in a medium saucepan, stir in the chopped leek, lemon juice, chopped basil and freshly ground black pepper, and serve immediately.

CARBOHYDRATE CONTENT PER SERVING: 2 GRAMS

Chilli and Ginger Sauce

For 4

2 tbsp extra-virgin olive oil
1 medium red onion, peeled and diced
1 garlic clove, peeled and chopped finely
2 slices fresh ginger root, peeled and chopped finely
2 green chillis, deseeded and chopped finely
1 tsp garam masala
$^1/_2$ tsp ground cumin
200 grams tinned plum tomatoes
1 tbsp tomato purée
freshly ground black pepper
1 tbsp chopped fresh chives
1 tbsp chopped fresh basil

- Heat the extra-virgin olive oil in a wok, and sauté the onion, garlic and ginger for 1–2 minutes.
- Stir in the chillis, garam masala, cumin, tomatoes and tomato purée.
- Season to taste, and heat gently for 5–6 minutes.

- Mix in the fresh herbs, and simmer for a further 2 minutes, then serve immediately.

CARBOHYDRATE CONTENT PER SERVING: 15 GRAMS

Chilli Tomato Sauce

For 6

2 tbsp extra-virgin olive oil
1 medium onion, peeled and diced
1 garlic clove, peeled and chopped finely
1 tbsp capers, drained and rinsed
1 small red chilli, deseeded and chopped finely
400 gram tin of chopped plum tomatoes
1 tbsp tomato purée
1 tbsp white wine vinegar
1 tbsp sweet sherry
pinch of rock salt
freshly ground black pepper
chopped fresh basil leaves, to garnish

- Heat the extra-virgin olive oil in a medium saucepan and sauté the onion, garlic, capers and chilli for 2–3 minutes.
- Stir in the tomatoes, tomato purée, vinegar and sherry, bring to the boil, then lower the heat and gently simmer for 20–30 minutes until reduced.
- Season to taste, and serve garnished with chopped fresh basil leaves.

CARBOHYDRATE CONTENT PER SERVING: 6 GRAMS

Basil Pesto Sauce

For 2

40 grams chopped fresh basil leaves
1 garlic clove, peeled and chopped
25 grams pine nuts, lightly toasted
25 grams Parmesan cheese, freshly grated
small pinch of rock salt
freshly ground black pepper
40 ml extra-virgin olive oil

- Add the basil, garlic, pine nuts, cheese and seasoning to a blender, and chop finely.
- Continue to blend as the olive oil is gradually added until a smooth, even consistency is obtained.

CARBOHYDRATE CONTENT PER SERVING: 2 GRAMS

Basil and Macadamia Pesto Sauce

For a delicious alternative to the traditional pesto sauce above, substitute the pine nuts with an equivalent quantity (25 grams) of macadamia nuts.

CARBOHYDRATE CONTENT PER SERVING: 2 GRAMS

Coriander Pesto Sauce

For 2

30 grams fresh coriander leaves
1 garlic clove, peeled and chopped
25 grams pine nuts
25 grams grated Parmesan cheese
pinch of rock salt
freshly ground black pepper
40 ml extra-virgin olive oil

- Add the coriander, garlic, pine nuts, cheese and seasoning to a blender, and chop finely.
- Continue to blend as the olive oil is gradually added until a smooth, even consistency is obtained.

CARBOHYDRATE CONTENT PER SERVING: 1 GRAM

Red Pesto Sauce

For 4

100 grams of semi-dried tomatoes with herbs
   (page 254), or jar of sun-dried tomatoes
1 tbsp chopped fresh basil
2 tsp chopped fresh oregano
1 garlic clove, peeled and chopped
1 tsp capers, drained and rinsed
2 tbsp lightly toasted pine nuts
1 tbsp red wine vinegar
80 ml extra-virgin olive oil
1 tbsp freshly grated Parmesan cheese
freshly ground black pepper

- Blend together the tomatoes, basil, oregano, garlic, capers and pine nuts in a food processor.
- Whilst the blending is continuing, slowly add the wine vinegar and olive oil.
- When the mixture is smooth, blend in the Parmesan cheese and seasoning.

CARBOHYDRATE CONTENT PER SERVING: 4 GRAMS

Satay Sauce

For 4

1 tbsp extra-virgin olive oil
1 small red onion, peeled and chopped finely
1 garlic clove, peeled and chopped finely
1 small red chilli, deseeded and chopped finely
3 tbsp peanut butter
100 ml coconut cream
$^{1}/_{2}$ tsp Worcestershire sauce

- Heat the extra-virgin olive oil in a small saucepan and sauté the onion, garlic and chilli for 1–2 minutes.
- Remove from the heat and stir in the peanut butter, coconut milk and Worcestershire sauce.
- Heat through over low heat, then pour into a ramekin dish.
- Cover and allow to cool.

CARBOHYDRATE CONTENT PER SERVING: 9 GRAMS

Capsicum and Basil Sauce

For 4

3 large red peppers, deseeded and chopped
1 garlic clove, peeled and chopped
1 tbsp chopped fresh basil
2 tbsp vegetable stock
pinch of rock salt
freshly ground black pepper
3 tbsp extra-virgin olive oil

- Blend together the peppers, garlic, basil, stock and seasoning.
- Add the purée to the olive oil in a small saucepan, and heat through to achieve a smooth consistency.

CARBOHYDRATE CONTENT PER SERVING: 7 GRAMS

Coriander and Basil Sauce

For 4

1 tbsp chopped fresh coriander
1 tbsp chopped fresh basil
1 tbsp chopped fresh chives
1 garlic clove, peeled and chopped finely
1 tbsp freshly squeezed lemon juice
1 tsp wholegrain mustard
pinch of rock salt
freshly ground black pepper
40 ml extra-virgin olive oil

- Add the coriander, basil, chives, garlic, lemon juice, mustard and seasoning to a blender, and purée.
- Slowly add the olive oil, whilst still blending, until there is a smooth consistency.

CARBOHYDRATE CONTENT PER SERVING: 1 GRAM

Barbecue Marinade

This marinade is equally suitable for meat or fish dishes.

For 2

4 tbsp extra virgin olive oil
1 tbsp light soy sauce
1 tbsp sweet sherry
1 tsp Worcestershire sauce
1 garlic clove, peeled and chopped finely
1 slice of fresh ginger root, peeled and chopped finely
freshly ground black pepper

- Mix the ingredients together in a medium bowl, preparatory to adding the meat or fish.

CARBOHYDRATE CONTENT PER SERVING: 2 GRAMS

Mango and Ginger Chutney

For 4

2 tbsp extra-virgin olive oil
$1/2$ medium brown onion, peeled and diced finely
1 large garlic clove, peeled and chopped finely
2 slices of fresh ginger root, peeled and chopped
     finely
1 green chilli, deseeded and chopped finely
     (optional)
pinch of ground nutmeg
$1/4$ tsp ground cinnamon
$1/2$ ripe mango
1 tsp caster sugar
3 tbsp Chardonnay
1 tbsp chopped fresh basil
2 tbsp freshly squeezed lemon juice
freshly ground black pepper
fresh basil leaves, to garnish

- Heat the extra-virgin olive oil in a medium frying
  pan, and sauté the onion and garlic for 2–3 minutes.
- Add the ginger, chilli (optional), spices, mango, sugar,
  wine and basil, and simmer on a low heat for
  3–4 minutes.
- Finally, add the lemon juice, season to taste, simmer
  for 2–3 minutes, and serve, garnished with fresh
  basil leaves.

CARBOHYDRATE CONTENT PER SERVING: 9 GRAMS

Caper and Basil Marinade

For 4

6 tbsp extra-virgin olive oil
2 tbsp white wine vinegar
1 garlic clove, peeled and chopped finely
2 tsp capers, drained and rinsed
1 tbsp chopped fresh basil
1 tbsp chopped fresh chives
freshly ground black pepper

- Add the ingredients to a screw-top jar and mix well.

CARBOHYDRATE CONTENT PER SERVING: NEGLIGIBLE

Cucumber Raita

Excellent for cooling the palate with a hot curry.

For 4

150 ml natural yoghurt
1 Lebanese cucumber, peeled, seeded and chopped
   finely
$1/2$ slice fresh ginger root, peeled and grated
1 tsp chopped fresh coriander
1 tsp chopped fresh mint
$1/2$ tsp ground cumin
fresh mint leaves, to garnish

- Grate the ginger with a ginger-grater.
- Mix together the yoghurt, cucumber, ginger,
  coriander and mint.
- Dry-fry the cumin, without oil, for 30 seconds, then
  add to the yoghurt.
- Stir well, and serve, garnished with fresh mint
  leaves.

CARBOHYDRATE CONTENT PER SERVING: 6 GRAMS

Coriander and Lemon Butter

For 2

1 tbsp chopped fresh coriander
1 tsp chopped fresh parsley
75 grams unsalted butter, softened
juice of a freshly squeezed lemon
pinch of cayenne pepper

- Mix together the coriander, parsley, butter, lemon juice and cayenne pepper in a medium bowl.
- Spoon into a ramekin dish, and cool in the fridge for 3–4 hours.

CARBOHYDRATE CONTENT PER SERVING: 1 GRAM

Horseradish Sauce

For 4

100 ml crème fraîche
1 tbsp grated horseradish
$^1/_2$ tsp caster sugar
2 tsp white wine vinegar
pinch of rock salt
freshly ground black pepper

- Blend the ingredients together, then chill in the fridge for 2–3 hours before use.

CARBOHYDRATE CONTENT PER SERVING: 2 GRAMS

Watercress and Mint Sauce

For 4

2 tbsp chopped fresh watercress leaves
2 tsp chopped fresh mint leaves
75 ml natural yoghurt
75 ml cream
1 tbsp freshly squeezed lime juice
pinch of cayenne pepper

- Mix together the ingredients of the sauce, cover and chill in the fridge for 2–3 hours before serving.

CARBOHYDRATE CONTENT PER SERVING: 4 GRAMS

Watercress and Mint Sauce (alternative)

For 4

Small bunch of watercress, chopped finely
1 tbsp chopped fresh mint
$1/2$ tsp Dijon mustard
100 ml crème fraîche

- Mix together the watercress, mint, mustard and creme fraîche, and chill in the fridge for 2 hours before use.

CARBOHYDRATE CONTENT PER SERVING: 3 GRAMS

Gravy

For 6

1–2 tbsp fat (from roasting tin)
meat juices (from roasting tin)
1 tbsp plain flour
250–300 ml stock
pinch of salt
freshly ground black pepper

- When the roast has cooked (meat or poultry), transfer the roast to a carving dish.
- Tilt the roasting tin, allow the fluid to settle for 10–20 seconds, then spoon off all but 1–2 tbsp of the fat which settles on top of the meat juices. This leaves the meat juices and 1–2 tbsp meat fat in the roasting tin – the basis for the gravy.
- Stir in a tbsp of plain flour until the mixture is smooth, then place the tin over a low heat and gradually add the appropriate stock (beef, lamb, chicken or pork, depending on the type of gravy), stirring constantly. The amount of stock to be added depends on the final thickness of the gravy, which is really a matter of personal preference.
- When the gravy is smooth, remove from the heat, season to taste, and serve immediately.

CARBOHYDRATE CONTENT PER SERVING: 4 GRAMS

Mint Sauce

For 4

2 tbsp chopped fresh mint leaves
2 tbsp boiling water
2 tsp granulated sugar
pinch of rock salt
2 tbsp white wine vinegar

- Mix together the mint and water, then stir in the sugar until it has dissolved.
- Add a small pinch of salt and allow to cool, then stir in the white wine vinegar.

CARBOHYDRATE CONTENT PER SERVING: 3 GRAMS

Apple Sauce

For 6

300 grams cooking apples, cored, peeled and sliced finely
3 tbsp water
1 tsp granulated sugar

- Place the sliced apple and water in a small saucepan and cook gently over a low heat until the apple has softened.
- Stir in the sugar until dissolved, and blend to a smooth purée.

CARBOHYDRATE CONTENT PER SERVING: 10 GRAMS

Index

ALSO AVAILABLE FROM VERMILION BY DR CHRISTOPHER GREEN

☐ **The New High Protein Diet**   0091884268   £7.99

☐ **The Ultimate Diet Counter**   0091889715   £3.99

☐ **The New High Protein Healthy Fast Food Diet**   0091894786   £7.99

FREE POSTAGE AND PACKING
Overseas customers allow £2.00 per paperback

ORDER:

By phone: 01624 677237

By post: Random House Books
c/o Bookpost
PO Box 29
Douglas
Isle of Man IM99 1BQ

By fax: 01624 670923

By email: bookshop@enterprise.net

Cheques (payable to Bookpost) and credit cards accepted

Prices and availability subject to change without notice.
Allow 28 days for delivery.

When placing your order, please mention if you do not
wish to receive any additional information.

www.randomhouse.co.uk